AN INTRODUCTION TO T'AI CHI

OPTIMA

AN
INTRODUCTION
TO T'AI CHI

ALAN PECK

ILLUSTRATED BY ALAN PECK

An *Optima* book

© Alan Peck 1990

First published in 1990 by Macdonald Optima
This edition published by Optima in 1993
Reprinted 1993

All rights reserved

British Library Cataloguing in Publication Data
Peck, Alan,
   An introduction to T'ai chi. — (Martial arts series).
   1. T'ai chi chuan
     I. Title   II. Series
   796.8'155

   ISBN 0-356-17220-1

Optima
A Division of
Little, Brown and Company (UK) Limited
Brettenham House
Lancaster Place
London WC2E 7EN

Photoset in 11pt Century Schoolbook by Leaper & Gard Ltd,
Bristol, England
Printed in England by Clays Ltd, St Ives plc

CONTENTS

PREFACE

T'ai chi chuan is becoming increasingly popular and, if
you want to study, it is becoming easier to find a class,
especially if you live in a town or city. There are a variety
of styles to choose from and within each style a teacher
will have his or her own individual approach, so that you
will probably find that one class is quite different from
another. But in spite of the variety of approaches there
are clear principles which are accepted by all t'ai chi
experts, and it is this fact which makes it possible to write
an introduction to t'ai chi chuan.

This book is intended for anyone who is curious to find
out more about t'ai chi chuan, because they are thinking
of joining a class. The outline of the history and meaning
of t'ai chi, together with a section on finding a class, will
help you to make an informed decision when you come to
choose a teacher to suit your interests. You will also read
something of what you are likely to find when you go to
your first class, and there are some guidelines to help you
with the learning. The stages of progress are mapped out,
starting from the beginning through to the more advanced
levels; even if you are already studying t'ai chi, you might
therefore find this a valuable reference book.

T'ai chi chuan has absorbed the attention of countless
people during its long history, and many different facets of
Chinese culture are revealed when you begin to practise. It
is as if you gain wisdom from the experience of practice,
without resorting to the written word or ideas from a book.
I hope that anyone reading this book may be inspired to
practise t'ai chi chuan and discover this for themselves.

Alan Peck

ACKNOWLEDGMENTS

I would like to thank John Kells and Dr Chi Chiang-Tao for sharing their knowledge of Yang style t'ai chi chuan with me.

Information on the Wu style was provided by Gary Wragg who is the Wu family representative in the UK.

My special thanks go to Justine Scott-McCarthy who patiently read through the manuscript and made many helpful suggestions.

1
WHAT IS T'AI CHI CHUAN?

Whether your first encounter with t'ai chi chuan is through watching a film about life in China, or from seeing it being practised in a less exotic location in this country, the slow graceful movements are instantly recognizable. A peaceful atmosphere and sense of stillness are apparent, providing a contrast to the frenzied rush often caused by the pressures of daily life. The movement is carefully performed and gives the impression of being coordinated and balanced, yet effortless at the same time.

The Chinese say of t'ai chi chuan that, if you learn the correct methods, you can gain the softness and flexibility of an infant, the strength and vitality of a lumberjack and the peace of mind and wisdom of a sage. This is so because the same principles of movement which produce t'ai chi chuan also influence our attitude of mind. Coupled with this sympathetic attitude, the postures liberate the subtle internal energy of *chi* to circulate freely around the body; this in turn makes the body flexible and builds inner strength. The system of t'ai chi chuan is different from the western way of thinking about exercise because it involves the body in a relaxed way, without using any force – the two key concepts which have made t'ai chi chuan famous.

ORIGINS OF T'AI CHI CHUAN

Towards the end of the fifth century AD, a monastery called Shaolin Temple was built in the Songshan Mountains of central China. Some years later it is said that an Indian Buddhist monk called Bodhidharma went there to teach Chan Buddhist meditation (the Chinese equivalent of Zen Buddhism) and he taught breathing techniques and physical exercises to complement the long periods of sitting in contemplation. Many of the eastern fighting arts, such as Shaolin, *karate* and *tae kwon do*, have been associated with these exercises originating from the Shaolin Temple tradition. They were based on the philosophical ideas of Chan Buddhism and in character and method have been called hard, external styles. The term hard has been chosen because force is used against force to produce impact, while the word external is appropriate because these styles apply the physical strength of the outer body. And in some cases a student will practise deliberately to harden the skin of the hands and feet.

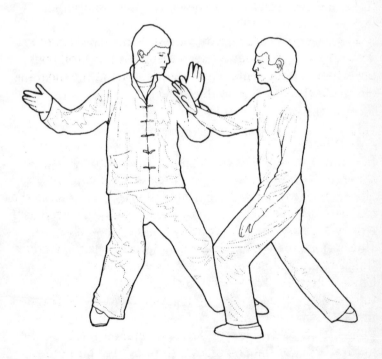

The t'ai chi master uses soft contact to deflect force without resistance

In contrast to this hard external style, there was a development towards soft internal systems using the ideas from Taoist philosophers and their particular understanding of nature. Here softness refers to the decision not to oppose force with force. For example, a master may step to the side as an attack is allowed to expend its force and then, as the attacker's balance is disturbed, immediately follow with a counter attack. The internal systems use the mind and sensitivity in addition to the subtle body energy called *chi*. There are three Chinese internal arts – *hsing-i, pa-kua* and t'ai chi chuan. Masters of *hsing-i* typically move in straight lines, with their strength coming down from above the head; it is a very direct method. *Pa-kua* favours circular steps with an emphasis on movement in the horizontal plane; it is evasive and subtle. T'ai chi chuan is the softest of the three and uses circular movements which function in every direction.

The concepts coming from ancient Chinese thought are very different from our western theories of natural law; nevertheless they remain an essential part of the meaning of t'ai chi chuan for us in the west.

BALANCE – THE ESSENCE OF T'AI CHI

In China almost everyone takes an interest in health; throughout their life they take care of their health and in old age retain much of their youthful vitality. In China the majority of t'ai chi chuan performers are middle aged or elderly because the rejuvenating effects are well known. However, in the west younger people are also attracted to this very enjoyable exercise, deeply embedded as it is in Chinese culture. The underlying logic of the Chinese theory of health is similar to the system of t'ai chi chuan; they both use the principles of early naturalist and Taoist thought, which explain the cycles of change and the natural order of the universe. If the way that situations and events constantly change can be understood, then it is possible to act in accord with the changes.

Consider a person who wishes to cross a lake against a head wind. They decide to use a rowing boat and battle their way against the wind to the other side. The going is difficult and they need a great deal of strength and effort to make any headway. Then, consider the same person using a sailing boat and sailing a zig-zag course to tack across the lake. The sailing boat is forced to take a less direct route to the other side because it is not possible to sail against the wind, although the sail is able to use the natural force of the wind to power the boat. The example of the rowing boat illustrates the use of the forceful, direct method which relies on brute strength; the example of the sailing boat uses the Taoist method, with a soft, yielding approach to harmonize with circumstances.

The Taoist approach dissolves much of the stress which arises from a struggle with difficult circumstances. One state changes into another just as, for example, day gives way to night. Later the cycle may be completed, just as night then changes back into day. The way to achieve health is thus to find balance and harmony within the changing facets of one's self; the varied individual aspects of the body and its functions are recognized as having qualities which should be balanced within the whole person. When stress is reduced in this way, the body's defences against illness are more efficient.

For t'ai chi chuan the whole body is relaxed to allow all the changes during movement to occur naturally. In order to relax thoroughly the body must be completely upright. The movements are balanced so that when going forward there is still the idea of going back, when bending down the idea of rising up is also present, and so on. During all the phases of movement in t'ai chi chuan the many meanings of balance become clear, and amid all the varieties of change a sense of stillness gradually comes to the fore.

It is helpful to learn something of the theory of t'ai chi chuan, and the underlying principles in order to build a complete picture of t'ai chi chuan, before becoming involved in the practice.

THE MEANING OF T'AI CHI CHUAN

T'ai chi means supreme pole, *chuan* means martial art.
The complete translation of t'ai chi uses the Taoist image
of the supreme pole; in 1173 Chu Hsi described it as 'That
which has no Pole! And yet [itself is] the "Supreme Pole".
It is the essence of that movement which produces yang
and that rest which produces yin ... all the many things of
the Universe go back to the one Pole.'

The two aspects of yin and yang represent the basic
dual division of things which we can recognize in everyday
life – light and dark, hard and soft, male and female,
night and day, etc.

THE SUPREME POLE

The 'supreme pole' refers to something like the apex of a
house or the ridgepole of a tent. This is the edge where the
two slanting sides of the roof meet at the top. From here
the two sides of the roof slope away and face in opposite
directions; therefore, when the sun shines on one side, the
other side is in shade. The light side is called yang, the
dark side is called yin. Yet these are not rigid divisions
since they are in constant flux as the sun traverses the
sky. The ridgepole is at the line of division and it is here
that there is an unchanging aspect amid the process of
change: this is t'ai chi.

Wang Tsung-Yueh in his writings on t'ai chi chuan says
'T'ai Chi arises from *wu chi*; it is the mother of Yin and
Yang. In motion they separate, in stillness they fuse.' *Wu
chi* is beyond concepts, pointing to the undifferentiated
raw nature of the way things are. It is often translated as
emptiness or as the void.

T'ai chi is the unchanging element that is within
change. It is similar to the axle of a wheel which remains
still relative to the movement of the rim. Or, to use
another image, t'ai chi is motionless and calm, like the eye
at the centre of a hurricane. T'ai chi gives rise to the
polarity of yin and yang and it is this polarity which

makes movement and stillness possible.

T'ai chi chuan embodies an understanding of yin and yang, the processes of change, and the stillness within movement. It reveals the different qualities of these opposites and the means to integrate them in order to find balance and harmony.

For the sake of convenience, t'ai chi chuan is usually abbreviated to t'ai chi. However, you should be wary not to confuse the philosophical concept of t'ai chi with the practice of t'ai chi.

WHO INVENTED T'AI CHI CHUAN?

It is generally agreed that there is no proof that any individual created t'ai chi. However the most popular, legendary story tells of Chang San-Feng teaching t'ai chi in the early part of the 12th century. Chang was also called Chang Lar-Tar, which means Sloppy Yang, because he was dirty and unkempt; whatever the weather, he wore only a monk's robe and always ate simple food. Chang was probably familiar with Shaolin internal exercises and boxing techniques, but he was a Taoist at heart and contemplated natural principles. It is said that he saw a crane attacking a snake and realized that the responsive loose movements of the snake were a good way to avoid the sharp stabbing actions of the crane's beak. Chang instantly realized the principles of t'ai chi chuan.

More reliable historical records show that Chen Wangting was practising and teaching recognizable t'ai chi principles during the late 16th century. Although before this date we can only speculate about the most likely beginnings, after this period the development can be traced to the present day. Today, variation and stylistic differences abound and there is no way to assess whether or not one system is superior to another or that one style has a better understanding of the principles. There are many benefits to be gained from practising any recognized style, since the essence is the same.

2
IS T'AI CHI CHUAN FOR ME?

WHAT DO YOU DO?

Although there are different styles of t'ai chi chuan, they all share many common characteristics. Basically there are three main kinds of practice for all styles – solo forms, partner forms and the use of weapons.

The solo form is a sequence of postures which link up with one another to form a continuous movement. Within each form there may be dozens of individual postures, as well as some repeated sequences. The forms are not standardized in the way they are put together or fixed in number, and if you compare each style you will find a considerable amount of variation. A typical short form will take from six months to a year to learn, and about 12 minutes to perform, while a longer type of form may take 25 minutes or so to perform. A student will gain the most benefit from practising the form on a daily basis.

All of the many partner forms use the principles of t'ai chi to harmonize with the oncoming energy of another person, as well as with the appropriate counter-responses. A fundamental idea is that force should not be applied against force. Ideally the body and mind are completely relaxed so that there is little or no restriction to the movement. Instead of bracing the muscles and locking the joints to develop a rigid type of strength, the t'ai chi habit is to do the opposite. There is a feeling of openness and the joints are never fully extended. The use of strength begins at the point of contact with the ground, coming from the feet and using the whole of the body in a coordinated way, until the actions are expressed in the hands and the entire body becomes responsive. There are

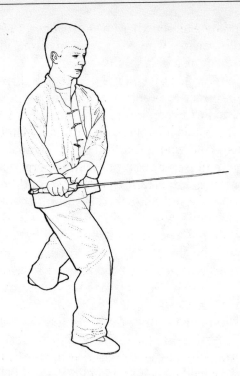

T'ai chi sword posture – push aside grasses to find the snake

many different types of partner forms; however, they can be simply divided into either those with fixed step positions or those with moving steps. The contact with a partner is generally sensitive and unlike other martial methods which use force.

The use of weapons in t'ai chi has been on the decline in recent generations, although the t'ai chi sword is still popular because its use is both graceful and quite athletic. It is still possible to find classes which teach spear and broadsword forms, especially within the Wu style.

CAN ANYONE STUDY T'AI CHI?

Yes. T'ai chi as a form of exercise is suitable for people of all ages, for both males and females, strong and weak.

With the guidance of an experienced teacher, t'ai chi can also be used by people who are recovering from illness or who have some physical disability.

Children enjoy the movements of t'ai chi, although they tend to find it easier to practise only for short periods, finding it difficult to keep interested and stay with one activity for the whole of a class. It is unlikely that a child under ten years old would find t'ai chi enjoyable, though, since younger children have a naturally energetic temperament; it is important that they should be free to express this openly and not asked to inhibit themselves.

A woman may practise t'ai chi throughout a pregnancy and will find that the habit of relaxing and the improved flexibility she gains are a useful preparation for birth. During the later stages of the pregnancy it may be necessary to take short breaks to sit down and rest before resuming the practice.

T'ai chi is famous for its value as a form of exercise to counteract the stiffness of aging. There is no need to strain the body during any of the exercises or movements, and the emphasis placed on relaxation allows the joints to open in a gradual way. For the younger student the approach can be different. If the steps are lengthened and the lower movements are developed to reach the deepest positions, then the whole practice becomes more physically and mentally demanding.

In the end it depends upon the student, for there is no one way of practising which is suitable for everyone. A student will find an approach which is challenging for them on a personal level while not being overdemanding. With the help of the teacher, a student can learn to avoid using force to attempt movements which put unnecessary strain and stress on the body.

MUST I BE FIT?

No. If you are unused to regular exercise it is easy to start t'ai chi with gentle movements, and then learn how to develop some strength and fitness later on. Perhaps the concept of fitness is becoming less appropriate for most people than the idea of achieving a general feeling of well-being, with mental as well as physical strength and resilience. T'ai chi is not competitive and there is no need to compare yourself with anyone else, since everyone is concerned with feeling how the principles of t'ai chi relate to themselves. For example, if there is a posture which includes turning the hips, then a student will feel how far the hips turn without using force. As this limit is approached, the turn is complete. As part of the early study of t'ai chi you will become aware of the internal experience of movement, and learn how to avoid using excessive strength. By studying and practising t'ai chi you will gain self-knowledge and self-discipline, which is ultimately more satisfying than the feeling of knowing more, or being more accomplished, than someone else.

So, you do not need to be fit to study t'ai chi. Indeed, if you are overweight, t'ai chi can provide the right kind of activity to keep you well exercised, and may be used as part of a weight-loss programme. Alternatively, t'ai chi will help build muscle if a student wishes to improve general health and develop some strength.

An experienced teacher can help a weak or sick student tailor their t'ai chi to regain their vitality. There are many stories of students who began t'ai chi to improve their health and then became masters themselves.

WHY START T'AI CHI?

As it is possible to approach t'ai chi in many different ways, there are various reasons for taking up a class. Perhaps the most common answer given is the desire to learn an art which will help relaxation and develop a peaceful frame of mind, while at the same time exercising the body. Other people say that they have seen someone practising t'ai chi and are attracted to the slow graceful movements.

Many are drawn to the gentleness and sensitivity of t'ai chi; as a form of exercise it is deceptively effective.

Although there is so much emphasis on relaxation with t'ai chi, with the exercise being performed slowly, the body weight is carried with great control and often balanced upon one leg at a time, giving good exercise to all parts of the body, especially to the legs. T'ai chi can be considered a unique form of exercise because it does not use one set of muscles pulling against another; the t'ai chi expert coordinates the movement of the entire body from the ground upwards, using the ground as the point of leverage and so permitting all the muscles to act in unison. Coordination improves with practice, and students will begin to feel more in touch with themselves as they learn how to use the whole body.

An interest in Chinese ideas and principles of living inspires many people to study. For example, t'ai chi can be used by an individual to raise their level of consciousness; the awareness is turned inwards and, as sensitivity becomes heightened, a more subtle awareness and presence of mind begin to mature. This is the basis for new ways of relating to the world. Others are curious about the system of developing internal energy or *chi*.

The martial art aspect is also often a factor for beginning to study t'ai chi, but this approach tends to be neglected since there are few teachers who understand the correct way to use the techniques. Even if the self-defence meaning is understood by the instructor, unfortunately it is seldom emphasized.

Perhaps the most common reason for taking up t'ai chi and practising on a regular basis is to improve health and vitality. It well deserves its reputation as a complete system of exercise for both mind and body. Many people take up t'ai chi without realizing there are more esoteric aspects to the exercise, gradually becoming aware of these underlying principles as they progress beyond the first stages of practice.

THE BENEFITS OF PRACTICE

Books on t'ai chi often stress its beneficial effects for

improving health. It is particularly helpful for building strength, the circulation is also improved, blood pressure is lowered, breathing gradually becomes deeper and this increases the efficiency of the lungs. The posture is improved as you begin to relax and feel the alignment of the body in every upright stance. Concentration and the ability to express the will are developed and, combined with the use of internal energy, this begins to improve general vitality.

An important benefit for everyday living comes with t'ai chi's influence on the mind. From the start the student learns to relax the limbs, and this grows into a habit, allowing the body to release the held stress in the muscles which for so long may have been in tension. Where there is stress there is also the tendency to hold on tightly. For example, if a person is absorbed in some stressful act the breath is sometimes held in quite unconsciously. During the time spent deciding to relax, the body gradually learns to feel that it is letting go of that held tension. It is only possible to relax the body completely when the spine is aligned with the forces of gravity and the body no longer leans in any direction. If, for example, the body tends to incline forwards, the back muscles must hold the body in tension to prevent it slumping forward and the weight moves on to the front of the feet, causing the toes to clench. Adjusting the posture and beginning to let go of muscular tension allows you to feel the body being more comfortable and open. Although this is mostly expressed in a physical way, it is the mind which is learning to let go.

But the mind can only relax a certain amount before there is a need for some kind of philosophy to help cope with the stressful situations one naturally encounters every day. It is of little use to be able to relax only when the conditions are ideal. So t'ai chi embodies a way of relating to changing circumstances, stressful or otherwise, and still remaining centred, responsive and relaxed. T'ai chi can be thought of as a form of meditation because it is a direct expression of Taoist philosophy; when learning t'ai chi a person is, at the same time, learning to harmonize with the natural order of the way things are (the Chinese natural philosophers call this The Tao).

The development of internal strength comes with the understanding of *jin*. This way of using the body does not use ordinary muscular strength. You might well ask how it is possible to be strong without muscles. It is not that the muscles are not used at all, but when the body is relaxed and the correct t'ai chi principles are used during movement, the *chi* begins to support the muscles. The mind directs the *chi* and, together with the supported muscles, the body behaves as if like a wave. The strength can flow, or pulse suddenly – this is soft *jin*. The t'ai chi master can also make the body hard at will. It is said that ultimate hardness results from ultimate softness. (*Jin* will be explained in more detail later.)

WHAT IS *CHI*?

There is no one word which can echo the meaning of *chi*. It can mean air or energy, but these words do not go very far to give any clear impression. Sometimes it is translated as breath. It is a good idea to settle for a general definition and keep an open mind until you have some experience for yourself. It is important to find a teacher who is familiar with *chi* and can demonstrate its use in t'ai chi, otherwise it will remain a mystery. It is helpful to contemplate the ancient Chinese scientific view which does not see matter and energy as separate. *Chi* is matter on the verge of becoming energy, or energy at the point of materializing. *Chi* can be felt in the body as a movement of energy; it may feel like the flow of an electric current, or the sensation of heat. In certain circumstances it can be compared to a magnetic force.

Chi is a very important phenomenon for the Chinese. Their knowledge and understanding of its use has steadily grown, but they do not try to explain it, instead observing its character and noting its behaviour. A Chinese t'ai chi master will not be able to explain how *chi* works, and will probably consider that such a question is unimportant.

There are 12 major pairs of *chi* channels and eight extra *chi* vessels. The 12 channels, or meridians, supply energy to the internal organs. When the *chi* is flowing smoothly the organs function as they should, but if the flow is disturbed and irregular, then there is a corresponding disturbance in the organ concerned. It has been said that the 12 main meridians constitute the rivers and the eight extra meridians constitute the reservoirs which absorb the excess energy from the main meridians. Of the eight extra meridians there are two which are thought to be major channels – the governing vessel and the conception vessel. These two channels are used throughout Chinese Taoist yoga and t'ai chi chuan. The *chi* is directed from the base of the spine, up to the top of the head, and then down through the roof of the mouth, connecting via the tongue with the front of the body and to the lower *tan tien.*

There are three main categories of *chi*: original *chi*, also called prenatal *chi*, which is transmitted from the parents to their children; grain *chi*, which is extracted from food;

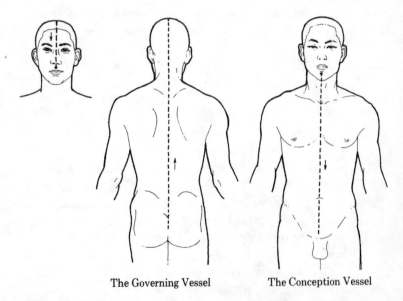

The Governing Vessel   The Conception Vessel

The two major channels – the governing vessel and the conception vessel

and natural air *chi*, which is drawn from the air we breathe. Within the three categories there are over 30 different recognizable types of *chi* which carry energy to the cells and organs throughout the body, some even extending beyond the physical body.

THE MAIN PRINCIPLES OF T'AI CHI

As already explained, t'ai chi is an internal system – the *chi* supports the coordination of the whole body, using the strength which is channelled through the joints, tendons and ligaments. In Chinese this method is called developing *jin*; it is often translated as internal strength, or whole-body energy. The principles of how to cultivate *jin* and its use are at the heart of all t'ai chi styles and forms.

The muscles are used, of course, but there is a feeling of letting go through the length of the body, through the feet and into the ground. This is called developing a root. In the early stages it is brought about by relaxing with the

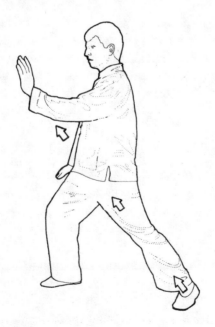

Brush knee and push

knees bent, letting the sense of self move from the upper body and settle below the navel area at a point called the lower *tan tien* (three finger-widths below the navel). The stability of the whole body is transformed as the feeling of relaxation moves first into the legs and finally into the feet. When the *chi* has been excited and mobilized in the body, and the relaxation has reached a complete stage, the *chi* sinks first to the *tan tien* and also into the feet. At this point the t'ai chi master is able to use a light and active connection with the ground and yet retain the ability to express power. It is important to have the feet rooted in this way so that a turn of the hips, when yielding to an oncoming attack, comes from a stable base. In a similar way, power during an attack is only achieved if there is sufficient leverage coming from the ground. The martial application of t'ai chi becomes a possibility when this level of progress stabilizes and becomes instinctive.

For the improvement of *jin* there are two most characteristic principles. First, there is never any use of force to overcome resistance, and second, all the movements are rooted in the feet and expressed through the body into the hands, elbow, shoulder or foot.

At first a teacher will guide you to use the body in a coordinated way and allow relaxation to become a habit. T'ai chi is considered to be natural movement, so it comes as a surprise to find that some of the positions adopted during practice of the form feel quite awkward and not at all relaxing. The reason for this is that most people have already formed habits which hold the body in a state of tension. During the early stages of learning t'ai chi the joints may be stiff and mobility restricted, but gradually, as the habit of relaxing becomes stronger, so the gentle exercise begins to undo the knotted muscles and unlock the joints.

After the movement has started in the feet, the energy travels through the legs, is gathered in the spine, and directed by a turn of the hips before it passes into the hands. It is said that the energy is expressed in the hands. The hips are important as the means of using the upper

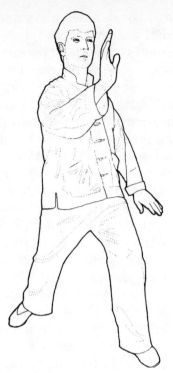

Yang-style posture – brush knee and push

body and coordinating with the arms without using shoulder strength; turning the hips gives the hands their direction. When soft *jin* is used, the body behaves very much like a wave, the energy unfolding from the feet and expanding into the hands. A push from the ground sends a pulse through the body to reach a concentration of energy in a small area such as in a hand or elbow; some masters also liken the action to the cracking of a whip.

After pondering on these examples it should become clear why the body needs to be so soft and relaxed – to allow the energy to pass through the body. This type of *jin* is the most obvious to the onlooker because it has a practical outcome, noticeable with powerful results when the t'ai chi partner is pushed. But there is another kind of *jin* energy which brings the *chi* to the surface of the skin and produces an unusual level of sensitivity, enabling the practitioner to detect the slightest movements of a partner. With practice this method evolves to the point where a t'ai chi expert can feel the flow of *chi* in another person. Initially there must be physical contact, but at a later phase it is possible to respond without touch, so that a master can detect another person's intention as well as feel the *chi* moving around their body. If a student practises to increase this sensitive type of *jin*, there is a general softening of the skin and the mind becomes keenly aware.

The tendons are used to express *jin*, while the muscle fibres are permitted to relax, allowing the *chi* to enter and provide support. The resulting strength is flexible and elusive. It can be withdrawn from an opponent's attack and then re-appear at a weak point. In motion the body is agile and light-footed; changes in direction are easily produced in order to follow the changes of adversary. The joints never lock and the limbs feel loose, but there is a clear sense of being connected throughout the body. The classics of t'ai chi say that the movements are like a great river rolling on unceasingly, and the postures of the t'ai chi form are connected like a string of pearls. If the muscles are used too much, then the *jin* produced is considered to be of a low level. It is the mind which needs to be made stronger and to be concentrated, for it is this which produces stronger *chi*. At first the mind is concentrated on the imaginary application of each posture; then the attention includes the *chi*, and coordinates with the application; later it is not necessary to pay attention to the *chi*.

MUST I UNDERSTAND THE MEANING TO REAP THE BENEFITS?

Yes. It is necessary to be aware of the meaning of the postures and their application to reap the full benefit of t'ai chi. The shapes of the postures are functional, and have self-defence applications. They become naturally strong when used in the appropriate way, and weak if they are used without this knowledge. From a t'ai chi point of view the posture is strongest when it is open and rounded at the same time, since the *chi* flows most easily if all the joints are held open and the shapes have a soft strength when they are rounded. This is similar to the strength of an egg, which can withstand a strong force compressing the two ends, but will crush easily when even a very weak force is applied across the middle.

It is important for the t'ai chi student, when choosing the most fitting shape for a posture, to have some awareness of the way it can be used, how the strength is released and in what direction. This knowledge is intellectual at first, but a student who has experience of practical use of a posture will begin to feel the strength directly. When the mind's intention is coordinated with the postures it should be in harmony with the strengths and weaknesses of the shape and at the same time express

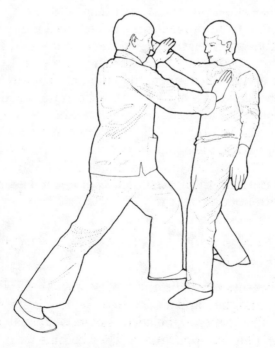

Application of brush knee and push

a sense of the imaginary use of the application. It is the mind's intention which leads the *chi*, and so for the *chi* to move the t'ai chi student imagines the application of the posture and acts out the function. The mind moves the *chi* and the *chi* moves the body. Without knowing the defensive meaning of t'ai chi, the mind is not involved and the *chi* has little power to move the body.

The benefits which t'ai chi brings for the inner mental well-being of a player are closely related to the imaginary world of shadow boxing. However, you may be interested in the health aspects of t'ai chi and not want to study the martial art meaning of the postures, perhaps because you do not wish to think of harming another person or to imagine that someone is attacking you. These are reasonable fears, and it is possible to find sympathetic teachers with more peaceful motives for practising the martial art application. The imaginary aspect of the form does not need to be given the shape of a person, as if each posture is a response to someone standing in front of you. It is possible to practise with a partner to get the feel of an application, and then to imagine the feeling of contact without thinking of attack and defence, but rather to feel a flow of energy coming towards you or moving away. The energy movement becomes the object which you feel and respond to.

EFFECTS OF T'AI CHI ON DAILY MENTAL HABITS

In the recent history of the west there has been a great deal of progress in the provision of material comfort, as well as advances in science and technology, making our lives more and more sophisticated. But many people now find they are so busy that there is little time to relax and be peaceful; consequently this need to relax becomes ignored. Yet material wealth does not solve emotional and mental difficulties, and so mental well-being is gradually becoming recognized as an important part of our lives.

Release of tension, dealing with stress

Relaxation is an important feature of t'ai chi; many of the principles of movement in t'ai chi are intended to permit the body to remain completely relaxed yet still be able to function in an active way. These principles sometimes relate to the physical qualities of the body, but there are those which guide the mental attitude.

Dr Chi Chiang-Tao, a grand master of t'ai chi, has said that t'ai chi is not complicated or difficult, it is just that t'ai chi habits are the opposite of our usual way. When faced with force, usually we react as if startled and meet force with force; when faced with stress we usually tighten, becoming tense. The way of t'ai chi is to meet hardness with a corresponding softness, and to relax the mind and body in every circumstance. There is sensitivity to what is happening, such that it is possible to respond in a measured way and act without conflict and struggle. Sensitivity increases when a student becomes openly more receptive.

The process of change begins with a feeling of acceptance and a sense of allowing events to evolve. This is a kind of antidote to the attracting force of rejecting something. For example, try not thinking of bananas. The more you try not to do something the more you are attracted towards it. So, if you wish to relax but notice some tension, perhaps in a shoulder, it is important not to reject the tension or try to make it go away. First there needs to be a feeling of acceptance of the tension, and an attitude allowing it to be there; during this mental process the tension will begin to dissolve.

Anxiety feeds on fears about events and situations which have not yet happened. We have a natural inclination to exaggerate the difficult and uncomfortable aspects of some things and the good qualities of other things. Our minds have the power to colour our experience in very convincing ways. There may be a dread of something which we think might happen in the future; but when the time comes we discover the real experience is completely different from our expectations. Nothing remains quite the same after investigating it more carefully. A coiled rope in a dark alley may appear as a dangerous snake lying in wait for us. T'ai chi brings a student more in touch with the way things are in the present moment, by learning to remain open and slow to judge – to live in the present and to value being aware.

Developing the will, learning to be flexible

If we face an obstacle which stands between us and the achievement of our aims, we search for a solution and hope that it will solve the problem. Even if the solution is not the right one, our instinct is often to keep sticking with it and simply to try harder or use more force. Sometimes this is the only option which seems available to us, even though we may have narrowed our vision of the problem too early and seized upon a solution that may be inappropriate. But we are committed and seem bound to stay with our chosen course of action.

The t'ai chi approach encourages an open state of mind which does not pre-judge a situation or jump to conclusions, allowing you to become more patient and to feel less hurried. It is possible to be quick without feeling hurried when the mind is clear and decisive. Through practising t'ai chi the mind is able to focus without being distracted by outside disturbances or internal mental chatter. A state is reached of total absorption in whatever you are doing, like a young child playing in an imaginary world without thought of anything else. The comparison with a child at play is useful, because a child does not become serious and stern when concentrating. There are no frowns or strains and the play itself is absorbing, as well as seeming lighthearted. As concentration becomes stronger, and you are able to focus more clearly on what is happening during the practice of the form, so the mind begins to feel uncluttered, lucid and free. When the thoughts become more directly connected to action and you are more aware of being in the present, then it is easier to be decisive. A conscious decision is made to listen carefully to, and be aware of, what is happening, and then to respond, all the while remaining open and prepared to adapt and change as the situation unfolds. Many students begin to feel more confident because they have learnt to be assertive and yet have not lost awareness, and are sensitive to how they relate both to others and their own situation.

Practising t'ai chi strengthens the willpower. At the same time it avoids the tendency to become too easily determined upon a fixed course of action, since the qualities of sensitivity and flexibility of mind are equally important. Gradually you can begin to understand the cycles of change by practising t'ai chi with a partner, learning to recognize that any oncoming force will have its maximum strength and then begin to decline. There is no need to deal with situations when they are at their most troublesome. The Taoist sage Lao Tzu recommends that we tackle difficulties when they are easy, accomplish great things when they are small and deal with a dangerous situation when it is safe. To see events clearly there needs to be an attitude of open acceptance, which is free from the tendency to interpret things in our own particular way.

DOES T'AI CHI CONFLICT WITH OTHER SPORTS?

The famous master Cheng Man-Ching is reported to have told his pupils that all sports are acceptable except skiing. The reason he gave for this one exception was that the possibility of breaking a leg was too great for him even to contemplate taking up the sport. Generally, however, there are no sports which cannot be combined with t'ai chi. The mental attitude of the player can become tense in some sports or too competitive to be consistent with t'ai chi principles, but this does not mean that you cannot change your mental game. Success depends upon playing a game well, and the quality of your game can be enhanced by t'ai chi. Balance and coordination improve from practice of the form, and speed of reaction increases as you relax, enabling footwork to become quicker and the ability to change direction to get better.

A fitness programme would not be contrary to t'ai chi if the student was mindful of the need to be relaxed and was able to avoid forcing the body excessively. Swimming, walking and cycling are all examples of compatible forms of exercise, but there are subtle adjustments which you can be aware of. If you consider cycling, for example, it would be important to avoid making the ankles tense by applying too much force through the ball of the foot during pedalling. The simple remedy would be to push down on the pedal from the middle of the foot.

Most of the beginning stages of t'ai chi do not exercise the lungs to any great extent and so an active exercise can be very beneficial, especially for a beginner.

IS T'AI CHI A FORM OF MEDITATION?

Yes. The whole activity of studying and practising t'ai chi directly affects the consciousness of the student. But unlike many other kinds of meditation, t'ai chi brings meditation into everyday life. The Taoist natural philosophy of living is expressed through the principles of t'ai chi. This is, in essence, a way of bringing together all the separate elements which we fix upon in our ordinary experience of the world and to blend them into a more realistic total-way of seeing. The Taoist would explain this as the balancing of the opposites of yin and yang and finding harmony with the processes of change, to become one with the Tao or the Way of nature. Scientists are now more willing to recognize the unordered chaotic way that some events happen in the natural realm and admit the limits of their ability to predict what is going to happen next. It is not possible to explain everything in a linear fashion since we live in a non-linear world and there are so many factors influencing any one event. In other words, we need to look at the whole picture to understand what is happening because everything has a bearing on everything else. T'ai chi helps an individual to expand his or her consciousness, in order to have more of the feeling of being a part of the whole; it is a truly holistic meditation.

The t'ai chi student is encouraged to become more open, with an expanded awareness. The openness is expressed in the way that he or she has no preconceptions or expectations about how any situation might or might not develop; there is a sense of being in the present and being able to respond as circumstances change. It becomes clear from practising t'ai chi that there is little need to be tense or to try to anticipate what is going to happen next. The t'ai chi master is able to expand his or her awareness to be conscious of many things simultaneously – this kind of attention is unfocused and spread over a wide area. It is similar to using the eyes with an unfocused gaze and being able to take in a wide scene in one glance; there is a more total vision. T'ai chi principles help the student use this heightened perception to observe change in daily life, to experience insight into the ways of achieving harmony and, in this way, to accord with each turn of events.

IS T'AI CHI TOO PASSIVE FOR MODERN LIFE?

No. T'ai chi is a useful antidote to the stressful pace of living, making it easier to remain calm and preventing the build-up of irritable states of mind.

Although t'ai chi promotes a very relaxed state of body and mind, it is important to understand that this does not accord with the usual image of someone relaxing – feet up, slumped in a soft armchair, dozing off to sleep with little motivation to move a muscle. An experienced t'ai chi expert will be relaxed, but his or her state of mind will be alert and the body will have the characteristics of activity. With regular practice you can create this balance between a relaxed stress-free state and a level of alertness and presence of mind which empower activity and the ability to get things done.

The Taoists observed nature and they believed that it was beneficial always to act in accordance with natural laws; they named this approach *wu wei* or non-action. This does not mean doing nothing and keeping silent, or letting everything take its course without interfering, but rather that every action should be appropriate and avoid using excessive force. It is in the Taoist's mind to seek balance and harmony between the dualistic ideas of yin and yang. This balanced state is called t'ai chi.

To gain the wisdom of a sage the principles of t'ai chi are contemplated in everyday life. The t'ai chi student begins by coordinating every part of the body until there is complete unification of movement from foot to hand, in every action. Following on from this, the mind's intention is trained to lead the body by acting out the applications of each posture so that the mind is then coordinated. At this stage, if the student is sufficiently relaxed, the *chi* will begin to be clearly experienced and then coordinated with the mind. Throughout the progressive stages of coordination the whole-heartedness of the student will be developed naturally as the awareness and concentration improve. Finally, the student reaches a more complete sense of being when the mind and body are integrated. It is then up to the student to apply what has been learnt on a personal level to experiences outside t'ai chi. Little by little, life becomes more like t'ai chi and t'ai chi becomes more like daily life.

3
THE T'AI CHI CHUAN BASICS

The Yang style is one of the most popular styles of t'ai chi; so much of what follows relates specifically to that style, although at the same time there are clear parallels to be drawn with other styles.

Although there are several different types of t'ai chi practice, in your first class you are most likely to begin learning some preparation exercises, followed by either the short form or the long form.

PREPARATION EXERCISES

Most t'ai chi masters practise a series of exercises before beginning the practice of the form. These are usually either to focus on one particular feature of t'ai chi practice, such as learning to direct the upper body movements from the hips, or to open the joints and release the stiffness in the body. There may also be a series of Chinese health exercises incorporated into the routine.

All of these exercises are recognized as a part of t'ai chi, and so are practised with the same relaxed frame of mind as you perform the t'ai chi form, without the need to use force to stretch the muscles. The advantage of practising specific t'ai chi exercises is that they are repetitive and make it possible to contemplate more subtle experiences of movement. For example, an exercise practised by some of Cheng Man-Ching's students begins with a fixed step position for the feet and a shifting of the weight to and fro. The arms are allowed to hang from the shoulders, and complete freedom is given to permit the arms to swing with the rhythm of the movement. At first you will find it a challenge to let go of the arms and leave them free to follow the motions of the body, but during the repeated cycles of the exercise, with opportunity to experiment, the imagination finds ways to give up the tendency to hold on to and inhibit the swing. It is possible to connect with the actual weight of the arms and decide to let that weight hang from the shoulder joint. Most of us do not realize how heavy the arms are because the shoulder muscles have been tense and in the habit of restraining their action; if you do begin to allow the arms to feel gradually more and more heavy, you will find that the muscles will relax and the arms will hang more freely. This method can lead to dullness and so should be balanced with an exercise which cultivates a feeling of lightness.

Another exercise looks like stretching and bending over to touch the toes. However, using t'ai chi principles, the body is completely relaxed and the folding action at the hips happens naturally as you allow the force of gravity to lower the body into a position where it is possible to touch the ankle. There is no force used to make the contact between hand and ankle. This is an effective way to loosen the hip joints and exercise the spine.

The health exercises are both numerous and varied. Some Chinese exercises are quite forceful, as well as strenuous, and should be avoided if you want to develop soft strength. Any exercise which sets one group of muscles pulling against another is not using t'ai chi principles; the body should function as one unit with every part open and relaxed.

There are also various gentle massage techniques applied to vital areas of the body. Rubbing and drumming points on the head are used, such as around the eyes to improve eyesight or at the back of the neck to relieve tension and improve hearing. The sinuses at the front of the face on either side of the nose can be stimulated to take away congestion. The kidneys are usually massaged with the back of the hand, using gentle but firm circular motions, and the front of the body around the stomach area can be given a massage with large rotations of the

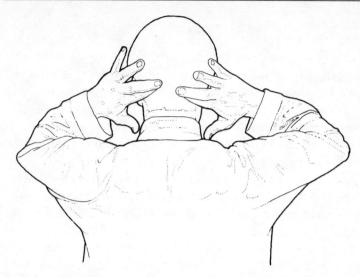

Drumming on the back of the neck with the fingers

palms to reduce stress and distribute excesses of *chi*.
These examples illustrate the type of exercises you are
likely to come across when you join a class. They can be
practised every day as part of your t'ai chi practice or as
part of a separate health routine.

Some exercises have been invented by masters to help
relax and loosen the joints or to improve the level of
fitness in a student. One example, invented by Dr Chi
Chiang-Tao, is described by him as dropping 'like a
sweater'. From a fixed step position you stand for a
moment with the legs slightly bent, and then flop down
with the hips loosening to let the seat drop, as if about to
sit down, but stopping just short of the ground. The whole
body lets go and flops into a low posture, like a sweater
dropping on to the ground – soft and loose. This type of
exercise encourages an open state of mind as well as
helping the joints to soften and articulate more easily.

Other exercises are aimed at reaching specific parts of
the body such as the spine, or the legs and hips. There are
areas of the body where the *chi* will flow more easily if
there has been some preparatory exercise; the back of the
neck and the lumbar part of the spinal column are obvious

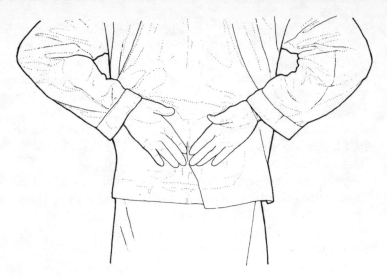

Massage of the kidney area

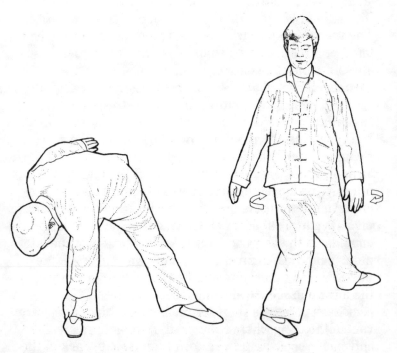

Preparation exercise

areas to focus on, because it is here that the *chi* tends to stick after the flow of energy has been increased during the practice of the form. The *chi* courses naturally up the spine from the sacral area of the lower spine, through the vertebrae to the top of the head, then down, through the roof of the mouth and the tongue, in front of the body, through the *tan tien* (an energy centre located two-and-a-half finger-widths below the navel) and back on to the base of the spine.

A sequence of preparatory exercises will take about 20 minutes to complete. If you do learn more routines than are necessary to fill your chosen practice time, then it is wise to vary the exercises you include rather than try to include them all every time you practise. If your time is short it is more useful to cut down on the preparation, and spend more of your time practising the form.

HOW DO YOU PRACTISE THE FORM?

The short form is literally a shortened version of the long form, and both are made up of a series of postures which link up to make a continuous practice. Each posture has specific martial art applications and, although separate from the next, flows on into the following one as if to make one uninterrupted action.

Cheng Man-Ching was a famous pupil of Yang Cheng Fu and he devised this shortened version of Yang's t'ai chi form for those people who did not have enough time to practise the longer version. He also felt that it was important to practise the form several times during a class to enable pupils to learn the form easily, and the longer form made this idea impractical. Cheng had some western pupils and did a great deal to popularize t'ai chi in the west. To give a flavour and a feeling of the movements of the form there follows a brief description of the first postures of Cheng's short form. You might like to record yourself reading this section slowly into a tape recorder, and then play it back so that you can concentrate on the following movements.

The first postures of the Yang style

To begin, stand with your heels together and the toes turned out. To help make the directions clear, imagine that you are now facing north. The legs are straight but not rigid, the knees are very slightly bent so that there is a feeling of looseness in the joints. The body is upright, with the sacral part of the lower back erect. The shoulders and arms are relaxed, the arms held at the sides of the body with the palms facing the sides of the thighs. The hands are relaxed and the fingers are held straight but not stiff. The head is balanced, neither slumping forward nor fixed too upright. The chin is tucked in a little, with the mouth lightly closed. The front of the body is relaxed, with some awareness of the *tan tien* region of the belly. Throughout this first posture all the joints, from the toes to the fingers, are allowed to feel open and relaxed. You should begin to

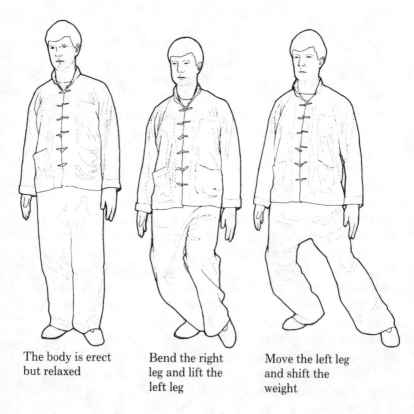

The body is erect but relaxed

Bend the right leg and lift the left leg

Move the left leg and shift the weight

be aware of the ground and the sensation of weight throughout the body, particularly in the feet. Experiment with a shift of weight and allow your centre of balance to move into the balls of the feet and into the toes; then move it back on to the heels. Settle the weight just forward of the ankle, and feel the upright balance in the body as you let go of any extra muscular effort you may have been using to counteract a tendency to lean.

Shift most of your weight into the right foot. Slowly bend the right leg to lower the body and, at the same time, lift the left leg from the knee so that gradually the left foot lifts off the ground, leaving just the toes lightly touching the ground. There is now no weight in the left leg.

Without disturbing the balance of the body standing on the right leg, reach over to your left (west) with the leg and place the foot with toes facing forward. Shift most of the weight into the left leg. The right foot is still turned out. Leaving the heel on the ground, lift the right foot and turn the leg, pivoting on the heel to bring the toes to face forwards. At the same time bring the arms away from the body; turn the arms to bring the hands around, with palms facing down and the fingers facing forwards.

The body now remains still as both arms lift together in front of you, the wrists loose and the hands hanging. When the wrists reach the level of the shoulders, the hands are raised level with the arms. Then the shoulders are loosened and relaxed as the elbows begin to drop down, bringing the hands in towards the shoulders, keeping the palms parallel to the ground. Before you bring the wrists too close to the shoulders and the arms begin to feel as if they are constricting the chest, allow the wrists to feel as if they have become heavy and are beginning to sink downwards, with the fingers lifted and feeling as if they are floating. The hands come down in this way in front of the body, and for the last part of the movement both legs bend to bring the body into a gentle sitting position. The weight is still mainly in the left foot.

These are the first two preparation postures of the form. There then follows a posture called ward off left.

Preparation posture, with fingers facing forwards

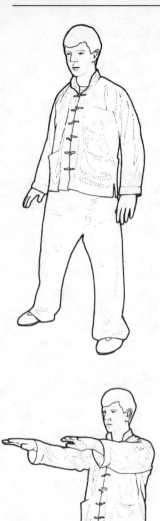

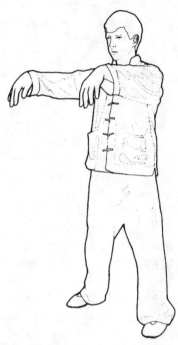

Arms lift upwards, hands hanging loose

The hands lift

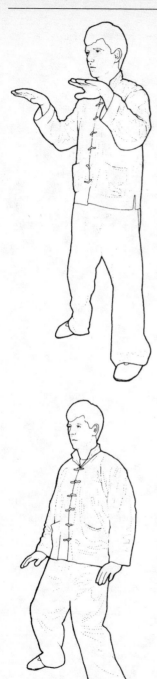

The wrists are drawn back towards
the shoulders

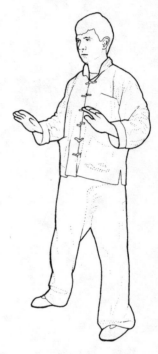

The wrists sink down, the fingers
floating

The body is lowered, coordinated
with sinking wrists

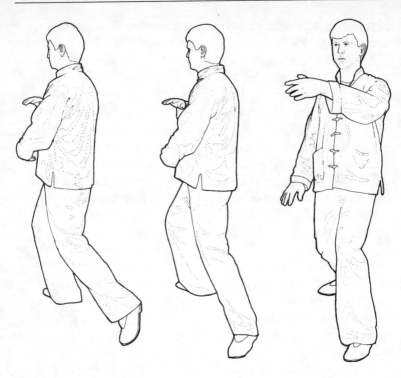

The hips turn right
and the weight shifts

The left leg steps

Ward off left
posture

With most of your weight still centred in the left foot,
turn the hips to the right to face east and, at the same
time, turn the right leg, pivoting the foot on the heel, and
bring up the right forearm with the palm facing down. The
weight then shifts into the right foot, and the left arm
comes across the body to bring the left hand under the
right palm, as if holding a ball.

The upper body and the hips now face west. The weight
moves into the right foot, and you then step north with the
left foot and shift the weight as you bring up the left arm,
away from and in front of the body, until the palm faces
the throat. The left arm is held in a rounded shape, with
the elbow lower than the wrist, to encourage a relaxed
shoulder. The right hand floats down and settles in front
of the right thigh. The waist straightens during this shift

of weight and the right foot turns slightly to follow the movement.

You have now completed the first postures of t'ai chi – and you may be feeling confused. It is in fact much easier to learn by following your teacher's movement than his words. When you learn the form you will become familiar with the principles of t'ai chi, and begin to get some ideas about how you can practise to achieve the benefits.

There are forms which include a weapon such as the double-edged *loong chuan* sword or the cutlass; these have the same kind of make-up as the short form. To take the example of Chen Wei Ming's sword form, this is practised at different speeds – sometimes slow and graceful and at other times dynamic and vigorous, with active steps and leaps. Usually weapon forms are learned after gaining at least a year's experience of practising the basic principles, or even much later when a student clearly feels the *chi*. The *chi* is moved to the end of the sword and maintained there, in the tip, throughout the whole form. The sword itself may be made from true sword steel, but finished without an edge, or alternatively may be carved out of a single piece of wood. The latter type would be used for partner practice to get the feel of attack and defence when faced with another person. The attack is aimed at the nearest part of a partner's body, which is usually the wrist if your partner is also wielding a sword; the attention must then quickly adjust to the counter attack after your partner has yielded and managed to avoid the blow. As a student of t'ai chi you gain a lively mind and quick reactions, as the attention must travel from your partner's body at swords' length, back to your own wrist, back and forth, with active steps as well as varied attacks. Agility and the ability to move in a fluid way are useful byproducts of this practice. Since the spirit of the contest is to help each other experience the use of the t'ai chi principles in action, and not to prove any kind of superiority, it is still relevant to keep to the t'ai chi habit of relaxing and never using force.

There are other partner practices which do not use any

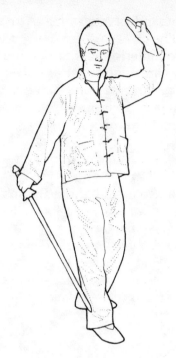

Yang-style sword posture – black dragon wagging tail

weapon, and these make up an important part of the t'ai chi syllabus. They are grouped together into two main areas of practice – those with fixed step positions and those with moving steps. In the beginning they are formal exercises to gain understanding of the basic techniques, using the principles of t'ai chi to deal with the oncoming energy of a partner. Later they become more spontaneous, are less restricted by form and the responses take on a much more instinctive character.

The different methods used in fixed step positions are single-hand pushing and double-hand pushing. These are simple routines, the form is easy to learn, and they are practised over and over again to acquire the right kind of sensitive touch and the habit of balancing and following a partner's force without being clumsy or losing any balance. There are further variations that have active moving steps, as well as slightly more elaborate forms, called *da lu*, which fit together with a partner practising the same form. The *da lu* postures repeat themselves as a never ending form, interlacing with the similar movements of a partner. The most elaborate exercise of this type is the Yang style t'ai chi dance, and continuous practice of this partner form gives a clear insight into t'ai chi self-defence methods.

WHAT HAPPENS IN PUSHING HANDS?

Pushing hands practice is not the aggressive sport you may imagine it to be. When you begin to learn the techniques you do not have to cope with someone trying to push you over, or attempt to push anyone else over; this is not the point at all. Pushing hands is an exercise designed to develop a subtle awareness of the energy and force of your partner, while maintaining perfect balance and

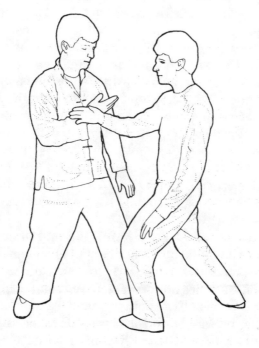

Pushing hands

equilibrium at all times so that the response can be perfectly coordinated. With this idea in mind, it is sensible to move slowly and sensitively during the early stages of training so that both partners can remain relaxed and aware of every movement as it happens and learn to apply the correct techniques. At a later stage of proficiency you would expect to be able to apply these same techniques to someone intent in pushing you over, but it is important to avoid practising with such a partner until you have acquired a firm habit of applying t'ai chi principles.

When you begin pushing hands you stand facing your partner in a formal position with one foot placed in front of the other; the distance between the feet should be similar to the width across the shoulders. The front foot is placed next to your partner's front foot, with your heel roughly adjacent to your partner's toes. You offer your forearm to your partner, who places his or her palm on your arm near the wrist. Your partner pushes your arm and you respond sensitively without resistance, moving the weight from the front foot into the back foot, whilst simultaneously turning the waist and gently turning your partner's force with your forearm. Finding no resistance, the force is spent and your partner's pushing hand is turned aside. The cycle is then repeated as your partner offers their arm and you move your hand to push your partner's wrist, coordinating your push with a forward shift of weight on to the front foot. There is more technique involved to turn the oncoming force, but this description is enough to give you an idea of what is involved.

Using weakness to overcome strength
Before you have learnt the correct t'ai chi technique there is a strong tendency to resist the force of a partner's push, even when this does not prove to be successful. If one person is stronger than another, then force can overcome the weaker person, but it is not possible to guarantee success every time; eventually you are bound to meet others stronger than yourself. It is, however, possible to

decide to be weaker than another person, and the t'ai chi method demonstrates how to be effective by using weakness instead of strength. In the hands of a good master this method can always be successful. To achieve a good level of competence with this technique you will need to progress through a number of stages, understanding the different ways of connecting with your partner's energy. There are four basic types of connecting energy:

- Touch is the simplest kind of connecting energy – the physical contact through touch.
- To stick is to keep continuous contact with a partner, which is maintained at the point of touch.
- When your partner moves, you follow whilst keeping sticking contact. If your partner retreats, you advance; if your partner advances, you retreat. If your partner moves quickly, you also move quickly; if your partner is slow you also choose to move slowly. Each action the adversary makes is mirrored with an appropriate response, without allowing any gap or separation of energy to open up.
- Finally, the fourth type of energy is joining. When your partner pushes you or tries to make a sticking contact, you feel their mind's intention, keeping contact yourself but preventing your partner from sticking to you. The t'ai chi master waits for the opponent to decide to move first, but responds before there is any physical expression of movement. This is the most subtle type of contact and requires careful practice to achieve the necessary level of sensitivity and coordination.

You will need to have these distinct types of contact demonstrated before it is possible to master them for yourself.

The value of training oneself to be sensitive and to avoid using force is realised when you discover that there is no need to have an attitude of resistance when faced with a potential struggle: it is possible to be accepting, open and relaxed. At face value it seems that t'ai chi encourages a very passive response to every problem, but this is not so; and there is more to the technique than just deciding to be weak and offering no resistance. On its own this solution would result in loss of balance and in being completely overcome by the oncoming force. When a t'ai chi master feels the force of an adversary, there is first a meeting and then a joining of the two energies, as the master follows the intended direction of the blow, introducing a deflecting energy of his own. It is this turning energy, applied at exactly the right time, at the appropriate point of contact and in the right measure, which is able to deflect even the strongest force away from its target. The master remains calm and relaxed, keeping a soft contact throughout the exchange, and the adversary is unaware of the neutralizing effect of the master's reply.

How do you turn an attacker's force?

Together with the passive idea of using relaxation, softness and weakness to overcome the force of an opponent, an active element is also introduced, just as the yin qualities are to be balanced with the corresponding yang attributes. The aim is to lead by following. The origin of this idea can be found in the ancient Chinese book of the *I Ching* or *Book of Changes*. This book was started more than 3,000 years ago, and many scholars and t'ai chi masters consider it as a source book for the ideas and principles of t'ai chi chuan. In the chapter on 'Following' it says that if you wish others to follow you, first you must be willing to take the lower position. So the t'ai chi master does not disturb the strength of the attacker's intended blow, and follows without resisting. At the same time, he attracts the force away from the body into open space by using a turn which uses the movement of the whole body coordinated with the *chi* and mind. The introduction of the circular deflecting force causes the original blow to be diverted, without the attacker having realized it. It is important to note that the attacker is not being blocked in any way, because this would rely on force applied against

force, and the attacker would be free to alter his or her
attack; the t'ai chi response leaves the attacker busy with
the attack, even though the blow does not meet its target.
It is this feature which t'ai chi exploits and which has
made it famous as a martial art.

What is the purpose of pushing hands?
If you study pushing hands for any length of time you will
begin to gain insight into the ways of using t'ai chi in daily
life. It is not possible just to read about t'ai chi philosophy
and then hope to convert that intellectual knowledge into
practical understanding. The reality of using t'ai chi with
a partner, and learning to avoid using force, gives a clear
perspective on the t'ai chi methods of releasing stress and
calming the mind. This results in your becoming more
sensitive, soft and aware – and of course it is also very
enjoyable.

When you learn the t'ai chi forms, your understanding
of the way to practise them is enhanced by your
knowledge of pushing hands, and vice versa. In the solo
forms you rely on your imagination to give meaning to
your actions, and these imagined responses are
remembered from practising with a partner. Pushing
hands gives you opportunity to put your relaxation to the
test and to discover the use of softness. When you discover
the effectiveness of t'ai chi and the practical use of the
principles, then you are encouraged to keep them in mind
during your daily life.

When we meet aggression we are all familiar with how
difficult it is to avoid getting caught up with our own
emotions, and then gradually to become aggressive
ourselves. If you can put t'ai chi philosophy into practical
use, then you can find more emotional stability and are
less likely to be drawn into uncomfortable states of mind,
such as anger or jealousy, and judgmental critical
attitudes.

MUST I PRACTISE ALL THE FORMS?

No. It is not strictly necessary to practise a complete range of t'ai chi forms in order to gain the benefits of t'ai chi. If you study the shortened form to a competent level, and have some knowledge of pushing hands, then you will be able to improve and develop your own understanding of the principles of t'ai chi. However, all the different aspects of t'ai chi do throw a different light on the essence of practice. It may be that you discover new ways of becoming dynamic and decisive by practising the sword form, which then inspires your shortened form practice. In this way you realize that different types of practice stimulate each other.

The complete syllabus is quite extensive, but there is no need to think that you should learn everything all at once. Developing a patient attitude and resisting the desire always to learn more is part of learning to relax and being present with one's experience as it is happening.

4
JOINING A CLASS

There are many books available which give detailed instruction about how to practise t'ai chi, using diagrams and commentaries, and there are videos which show the postures and explain the different points to be aware of when copying the form. Despite all that, it is not possible to learn very much without an experienced teacher who is able to demonstrate the feeling and attitude of t'ai chi and to teach the more subtle levels of meaning.

You may see t'ai chi classes advertised on noticeboards at local libraries, universities, clinics for alternative medicine, wholefood shops and restaurants, bookshops and other shops which display posters. Some cities have magazines with information about what is happening in the local area, and t'ai chi classes are often advertised in these.

Begin your search by finding out what is available, and then try to arrange a visit to an existing class, or telephone the teacher and ask for details about the type of t'ai chi being taught and the way the classes are organized.

The cost of classes will vary, depending upon who you study with and where the class is located. The cost of tuition in London with an established teacher can be between £5–10 per class, but classes organized by the local authority or in other parts of the country, may cost as little as £1 (1989 prices). There are usually no extra costs such as affiliation fees to an organizing body, and no uniform to buy before you begin your study.

FINDING THE RIGHT TEACHER

From the early years of development of t'ai chi up to the present century, the correct methods of technique have been kept secret within t'ai chi families. When a master was teaching his students it was traditionally accepted that if another t'ai chi expert came along, challenged the master to a contest and defeated him, then the master would give up his school to the victor and leave in disgrace. It is not surprising, therefore, that the master would be very guarded about his knowledge, even with his own students. Knowledge was handed down carefully from father to eldest son, and it is said that in some cases a father would wait until he was about to die before giving his secrets away. Sadly, this secretive oral tradition has been responsible for the loss of many techniques, and in particular those which develop the *chi* to the more advanced stages.

The circumstances have now changed a great deal; there is no need for secrecy, and the patriarchal barriers have been removed. However, some teachers still refuse to teach openly, they leave students' mistakes uncorrected, or even withhold information. In some cases this may be because their knowledge of t'ai chi is scant, or perhaps they had to make so much effort to break through the secrecy barriers themselves that they are now reluctant to make things easier for their students. Some teachers have much to say about the philosophical aspects of t'ai chi, and how to put t'ai chi principles into practice in daily life, and yet are not able to demonstrate even the first level of achievement in their own t'ai chi practice.

It is therefore important to learn to discriminate when deciding upon the right teacher. T'ai chi has never been regulated by an official organization, and so it is left to your own personal judgment to decide whether one teacher suits you better than another. There are, however, some pointers which you may find useful when making your choice.

In choosing a teacher you should first establish whether that person has received teachings from a recognized master belonging to a recognized style. Ideally it should be possible to trace back a line of successive teacher/pupil relationships going back to one of the more famous masters of the 1900s. The connection in itself does not

mean that the teacher has understood what was taught, or
that they had enough talent to master the teachings, but it
is an important start. Most teachers will be quite used to
being asked who their teacher was, and who taught that
teacher. Be careful to avoid those minor students who
have not studied with a master, or who have studied only
part-time, and yet set themselves up as instructors
(although it might be well worth studying with their
teacher).

It is a good idea to make sure that what you are
learning is pure t'ai chi, since some t'ai chi teachers have
studied other styles of martial art and may teach a
mixture of t'ai chi with some other techniques which come
from another distinct style. For example, it is not possible
to practise, or teach, hard and soft styles at the same
time, although it is quite common, and acceptable, for a
teacher to be teaching *pau-kua* and *hsing-I*, as well as t'ai
chi, since these are all soft styles.

THE DIFFERENT STYLES OF T'AI CHI CHUAN

There are three main popular styles of t'ai chi chuan –
Yang, Wu and Chen – and a few other minor styles. Li
style is indirectly derived from the Chen style, and Sun
style is indirectly related to Li style. All these names
relate to the original family names of the founding
masters, and although they are recognized as being
separate and distinct styles, they all have the same
origins.

After Chang San-Feng, the most famous masters of t'ai
chi included Wang Tsung-Yueh and Chiang Fah. It was
Chiang Fah who taught t'ai chi to the Chen family, where
it developed for 14 generations before dividing into old and
new styles. The old style was favoured by Chen Chang-
Shen, and the new style was devised by Chen You-Ban.
Chen Chang-Shen taught outside the family to Yang Lu-
Shann and Li Bao-Kuai. Yang Lu-Shann transmitted the
style to his two sons Yang Ban-Huo and Yang Chen-Huo,
and so the Yang style was established. Wu Chun-Yu then

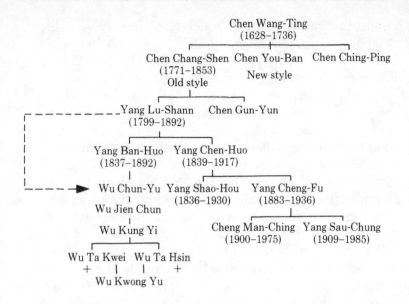

The family connections of the main t'ai chi masters of the Wu and Yang styles

learned from Yang Ban-Huo, and founded one of the Wu styles. The story is a complicated one, but in this simplified version it is clear that the different styles are intimately related.

Chen is the oldest of the modern popular styles. In the early forms there were many vigorous actions, such as leaping into the air and stamping, but these have been reduced in the more modern versions. The Chen style still retains very active characteristics, with dodging gestures, swift movements and some stamping of the feet. There are spiral-like turning movements, which alternate with extending and withdrawing actions, standing firm and then becoming soft, moving quickly and then slowing down. Chen style is much more dynamic than the other styles, and contains a whole variety of expression of energy.

By way of contrast, the Wu style is much more compact, with emphasis on the use of open and closed postures, employing small circles, with the idea of martial application having an obvious influence. Gary Wragg, the Wu family representative in the UK, defines the main internal emphasis in the Wu style as softness and sticking, which are also important characteristics for the Yang style. The Wu style movements have retained their compactness from Yang Lu-Shann's small circle style, and most of the postures are practised with the weight completely in one foot at a time, although the forms do include the riding horse stance which has the weight equally divided between the feet. Another distinctive characteristic of this style is the stretching back leg (the yin leg), which creates a type of elastic softness balanced by the firmness of the stance.

The Wu style is 99% use of the hips. The hips are loose and relaxed when turned and the spine is always straight whatever the posture. The hip and waist move together coordinating with the whole body. When a Wu style master uses the energy of the whole body, the leverage, coming from the feet, causes the waist to turn, creating a spiral action which then transmits into the hands.

The Wu style masters of the present day have descended from Wu Chun-Yu who taught his son Wu Jien Chun, who in turn passed his art on to his son Wu Kung Yi. He taught his nephew Wu Ta Hsin and Wu Ta Kwei who then taught Wu Kwong Yu. Wu Kwong Yu is the present day master of the style.

The Yang family style has been the most popular style of t'ai chi in recent years. Yang Cheng-Fu was the second son of Chen-Huo, and it was he who managed to find a way to teach his father's fine art to a wider community by simplifying the form and leaving out the quicker movements which had survived from their Chen origins. Cheng Man-Ching studied with Yang Cheng-Fu during the last part of Yang's life, and later became famous as an accomplished master, able to inspire many western students to study and practise t'ai chi.

Chen Man-Ching's form is slow, fluid and rounded, with postures which are comparatively easy to learn and

movements that do not require too much effort to
practise. These features have made the style popular with
many people from all walks of life.

Students of t'ai chi at the first level are described as
being at the level of using 'force against force'. Most
people, when they begin t'ai chi, out of habit will resist a
force coming towards them by using force themselves. You
should expect a teacher not to use any force in any of his
or her t'ai chi; all their actions should be completely
relaxed.

It has already been explained that it is important to
understand the use and application of the postures if they
are to be meaningful. So consequently it is a good idea to
make sure that your teacher has a complete knowledge of
how each posture is used in self-defence, as well as
knowing the different aspects of pushing hands.

There are many different reasons for taking up t'ai chi
– for health, as an antidote to stress, as a way of
approaching Chinese philosophy and meditation – and
you would be wise to find a teacher who is sympathetic
towards your particular motivation. A teacher who talks
about the philosophy at great length may not be very
involved in the practice of t'ai chi; if the classes are full of
strenuous exercises, then the soft aspect might be
neglected; and so on. Be aware of what benefits you hope
to derive from your practice before you seek out a teacher,
and then check to see if the teacher will be able to offer
the emphasis you want.

Beware of any personality cult surrounding a teacher,
especially if it is encouraged by the teacher. A good
teacher will treat you as an equal and it is only from such
a person that you will learn to be open and relaxed
yourself. However, once you have made your decision to
join a class, be careful not to be too quick to judge the
teacher, and try to learn with an open mind. If you have
too many expectations about how a teacher should be, you
are bound to be disappointed.

It is very important to have faith in the teacher, but at
the same time you should test the truth of his or her

advice by putting it into practice and coming to your own conclusions. Do not be too quick to accept teaching at face value. When you hear advice, contemplate the meaning, then put it into practice and be aware of the experience. Try to learn from the experience of your practice.

WHAT CLOTHING IS NEEDED?

There is no need to buy any special clothing for practising t'ai chi. Any loose fitting clothing which allows you to move with complete freedom is suitable. There is a traditional Chinese style of suit which you can buy from martial arts shops, but this is more likely to be worn exclusively by the teacher and senior students, so it may be a good idea to check before you buy one. Tracksuit trousers are ideal for giving freedom of movement, even during the more expansive positions of the t'ai chi form.

For the feet you will need light footwear which does not have a raised heel. There is a type of Chinese slipper, sometimes called a *kung fu* shoe, which is a good choice for t'ai chi. They are usually black with a variety of different types of sole. The rope sole version does deteriorate very quickly after getting wet, and may also be quite slippery. A better choice is the plastic sole which is hard wearing, and more comfortable than you might imagine, but may be a problem if the class is held on a polished, slippery floor surface. In this case there are kung fu slippers with rubber soles.

Some t'ai chi students do wear trainer shoes, but these can be too heavy and cumbersome for sensitive contact with the ground, and tend to make quick footwork awkward. If the floor surface is comfortable you can practise the beginning stages of t'ai chi in bare feet but protection for the feet is advised when you practise the faster techniques of more advanced stages.

WHAT CAN I EXPECT IN A CLASS?

A class for beginners may vary in size from half a dozen to

perhaps 25 individuals. It is a good idea to avoid classes larger than this because it is always important to have some personal contact with the teacher, and large classes tend to be over organized and impersonal.

There is no set format to a t'ai chi class, and you will find there are a variety of different styles of teaching. Some classes have a mixed group of students at various different levels of experience who are divided up into smaller groups and given instruction, one group at a time, and then left to practise whatever has been taught, perhaps with the supervision of a senior student. This method does not give you much time with the main teacher, although you may find it helpful to have the assistance of a more senior student who is able to share an experience of t'ai chi which is not too removed from your own. There is the advantage of learning at a leisurely pace, but it may be that you are left much more to your own devices.

Another way of organizing the class is to have all the students at the same stage of learning and to teach one posture or technique at the same time to the whole class. This method is quite efficient and the group has the full attention of the teacher throughout the duration of the class, so that practice is supervised and questions can be answered as and when they arise. The disadvantage of this method is that if you miss a class then it is easy to fall behind the rest of the group; you then have the difficulty of trying to catch up. If you choose a teacher who does organize his classes in this way, you can find out what help would be offered to you if you were to miss a class.

A class may vary in length, between one and two hours. There is no need to feel daunted at the prospect of spending a whole two-hour session doing physical exercise; t'ai chi is a relaxed and gentle system which avoids force, and there will be some variety of activity within that time.

A class is likely to begin with some preparation or health exercises, then practice of the form with some revision of the previous week's lesson, followed by the introduction of new postures or techniques. There may be some partner techniques practised as part of the class, or perhaps the teacher will suggest an exercise to help develop a particular aspect of t'ai chi. You may also be offered some refreshing Chinese jasmine tea at the end of your class, since this is the custom in many traditional t'ai chi schools.

Is there any tradition of etiquette?

There are some t'ai chi schools which expect their students to show respect for the traditions of the style by bowing at appropriate moments – usually before entering and leaving the class. You will find that different schools have different expectations of their students, and there is no general rule to guide your behaviour other than to be respectful, especially to the teacher and senior students. You will learn the appropriate etiquette from watching the behaviour of the experienced students, and the teacher will explain anything not immediately obvious.

Cheng Man-Ching said that it was important to help, protect, love and support the higher students. He said that there was a reason: 'The higher he goes, the higher he carries us.' There is mutual influence. As the more experienced students improve, so they influence all those who come into contact with them.

It is also very useful if you can show respect to all other living beings – to respect life itself – and develop the feeling that you wish every being to fulfil itself and achieve true happiness. This will encourage you to be open-hearted and counter any feelings of separateness and pride which will remain as obstacles to your own achievements.

HOW MUCH EFFORT IS INVOLVED IN T'AI CHI?

When you begin t'ai chi the experience is probably new and strange, but you will become more familiar with the t'ai chi way of moving and expressing your energy in a gradual way – the process takes time. You will find it helpful if you remember to approach t'ai chi in a relaxed way, and let your interest and involvement develop at its own natural pace. Studying and trying to learn in a class can be a tense activity, particularly if the pace of the class is too fast for you. However, it is not usually necessary to learn everything on first hearing, as there is likely to be a great deal of repetition.

T'ai chi is famous for relaxation, yet many people say that sometimes, when they have finished practising, they are more tense than they were when they started. Why is this? When you begin the form, standing in the attention posture, the mind can easily begin to tighten because you think 'Now I am doing t'ai chi' and unconsciously there is the feeling that this is something special and unusual. So, when you begin to move you are trying too hard and wanting too much. Learn to relax the mind by thinking of t'ai chi as something very ordinary, which you can approach in a casual way and yet still be careful. Another attitude of mind is to allow yourself to think that you are already a master and have the confidence to move in a very relaxed way without any fear of making mistakes.

IS THERE ANY DANGER OF INJURY?

T'ai chi is essentially a gentle activity; even when practising at considerable speed with a partner, the contact is soft and well coordinated. Unlike *aikido* or *judo*, there are no falls or rolls on to the ground. The body stays upright in all of the postures, including those with a squatting stance, and the improved sense of balance which is cultivated means that there are no extreme stresses applied to joints or muscles during any of the exercises.

T'ai chi exercises, operated together with changes in mental attitude, begin to affect the body and bring about small changes in the muscle and bone structure as you learn to relax and sink your centre of gravity into the belly and feet. If, for example, you have been hunching your shoulders and, through your t'ai chi practice, you manage to find ways to relax them, then pain may be caused by the muscles releasing the knots of tension. The collar-bone may move a little as the shoulders drop, which, until the body adjusts, can also be uncomfortable. Some people find that when the feet relax and the body's centre of gravity is balanced in the middle of the feet, the arch at the base of the toes, between the toes and the ball of the foot, can drop and the feet spread out to become flatter. These changes occur because the body is becoming more open, through the use of gentle, unforced exercise, and the changes are a quite natural healthy sign of improved posture. Although there can be slight pains associated with these changes, they are normally temporary and should clear within a week or so.

It is rare for anyone to sustain any injury during their t'ai chi practice, but there are some dangers which you should be aware of. Most of the postures involve turning the hips, and if the hips are stiff then this effort to turn can force the legs to twist rather than the hips to turn. The knee joint is very vulnerable when the leg twists and can be damaged. Care is needed to ensure that the waist and hip turn articulates the hip joint so that the knee is left undisturbed. You will notice that the knee stays aligned with the direction of the foot, showing that there is no twist.

The knee is also vulnerable to strain if you try to step while in a low stance without being sufficiently relaxed, or without taking care to keep the spine vertically upright. The stride should be long enough to need some mental effort when stepping, but not so long that you struggle to shift your weight and become tense during the step. The hips and the feet should always feel loose, even when they are carrying your weight. The danger occurs when the muscles around the knee have too much work to do on their own to give you the necessary leverage to lift the other leg. The safest way to take a step is to keep the body balanced and upright, shift the centre of gravity over the foot which carries the weight and only then, when the stepping foot is completely empty of weight, make the effort to step.

PHYSICAL WEAKNESSES WHICH CAN PREVENT STUDY

If the knees are weak due to some previous accident or injury, then you should rest from your practice until there has been a complete recovery. It is easy to aggravate a condition without realizing it. If you have other physical weaknesses your practice can usually be adapted around them, with some guidance from your teacher, and often you find that the exercises are beneficial. For example, t'ai chi is an excellent method of improving your posture; the use of strength comes from understanding your relationship with the ground, and it is possible to strengthen a weakened back through practising the form, as well as learning good habits for lifting and carrying heavy weights.

T'ai chi is about relating to your body as it is and becoming in tune with that inner experience so that you can find new ways of expressing your energy in a more natural way. Whatever problems you have to work with in your body, there need not be any serious restriction to your practice if you are able to find the way to adapt your t'ai chi while conforming to the principles. This is true for those who have physical disability and are not able to practise t'ai chi in the conventional way. An experienced teacher will be able to help you adapt the t'ai chi postures and movements to accommodate your particular difficulty, but you may need some individual tuition.

5
BEYOND THE BASICS

HOW MUCH SHOULD I PRACTISE?

Enthusiasm is a precious quality for the beginner, and you
should be careful not to use it up all at once by practising
too much too soon. However much you enjoy t'ai chi, you
will soon tire of it if you practise every spare minute, every
day. It is much better to practise little and often than to
practise for one long session once a week; 10 or 15 minutes
practising your preparation routine, and a further 10 or 20
minutes practising the form are good lengths of time to
begin with. If your mind wanders too often during the
session, then shorten it next time. If you decide to
practise, for example, 20 minutes on any particular day,
then finish your session when the time is up. It will help
your concentration and the development of your power to
be decisive to keep to the time you have chosen for that
day. The benefits of t'ai chi are accumulative, and so
regular practice is something to aim for. Do remember
that t'ai chi is intended to improve the quality of your life,
and not to become another problem for you; it is likely
that you have enough problems already.

If your practice is irregular do not despair or inflict
guilty feelings upon yourself; use the experience as an
opportunity to develop a relaxed attitude, and at the same
time think about the advantages and benefits of
practising, and so organize a definite time for your next
t'ai chi practice. There may be times when you do not feel
like beginning your practice session because you feel a
little tired, or feel generally low in spirit. This is a good
time to practise, since the form will open your mind and
body with an improved flow of energy which will influence

your state of mind positively and energize your body. However, if you do begin a session and your mind and body feel too tired, and there is a sensation of heaviness, with the head tending to drop forward, then it is a good idea to rest, otherwise you will be practising dullness. And there will be days when you have no time to practise, although if you have the opportunity to remember the feeling of t'ai chi, and think about being relaxed and soft in your daily life, this can be very beneficial.

A balanced attitude towards the content of your practice will also keep your mind alert and fresh. Vary the way you practise, as well as what you practise. For example, the first practice of the form should be completely relaxed, with little concern about getting it right. The next time you repeat your form, pay attention to the techniques involved; ask yourself if you are completely balanced before taking a step, whether the movements all originate from the feet, legs and waist, if the shoulders are relaxed and the elbows lowered, and so on. Practise individual postures to consolidate any corrections you remember receiving during your last class, and finally practise the form in a fluid relaxed way with a light sensitive attitude, to experience the joy of t'ai chi. Studying t'ai chi has its share of hard work, but it is important to remember to set aside some time for pure enjoyment.

The best speed to practise

During the early stages of study it is a good idea to practise slowly so that you have time to feel inside your body and experience your body states clearly, as well as being aware of coordination. It is much easier to relax if you give yourself plenty of time to let your body weight sink between each movement, pausing to feel your weight focused into one foot before moving the other empty leg. You should not feel that you cannot stop completely if you are unsure of your footing.

When you have learned the first section of the form you can experience some of the flow of the sequence by occasionally practising at a faster speed. However, by some standards even the faster speed would be considered to be slow, and so you should ask for guidance from your teacher.

How do I practise at home?

If it is possible you should practise in an open space, outside, preferably near the trees, where the air is fresh and well oxygenated. Of course this is not always convenient, although pleasant, and any clear space in your home will do just as well. If your room is not really large enough and the furniture gets in the way, be aware of not allowing this to intrude as a source of irritation. Although it is not ideal, you can practise sections of the form and then adjust your position before you restart your practice.

Some individual postures are suitable to be practised in isolation, but there are also those postures which will link up with each other and repeat as a series. You can use this type of practice at any time – perhaps whilst waiting for a meal to cook, or as a break from some other activity. It is a good idea not to be too precious about your practice; if you feel easy-going about t'ai chi you are much more likely to feel spontaneous about when you practise.

WHAT PROGRESS CAN I EXPECT?

Progress in t'ai chi is not measured in the same way as other martial arts; there are no grading systems or belts awarded, or certificates of achievement, because t'ai chi is not organized as a competitive sport. There is, however, a progression through a number of stages of development which have set features, although variously described by different schools.

The time involved in reaching a competent level depends upon three main factors; correct teaching, the pupil's ability and the persistent desire to practise. The most important of these is to receive correct teaching from a qualified teacher, because without this you may practise for years without making very much progress. Ability is not as important as you might suppose; if a slight amount of natural talent is balanced with a persistent desire to practise, then it is possible to make sustained progress and gain much from your practice. Also, it should be said that a talented person who is lazy will not gain much from their short periods of irregular practice.

The first year of t'ai chi chuan

Some of the results of practising t'ai chi will be felt within the first few weeks of beginning a class, but other benefits are felt only after the accumulation of regular practice, over a longer period of time. The rate of progress will vary with the individual.

In the first weeks you will find some positive benefit from making a regular effort to relax. This will be consolidated if it occurs to you to remember to relax during your daily routines and to approach other activities with a t'ai chi frame of mind. The centre of gravity will begin to drop as the tension in the upper body is released, and you become increasingly able to coordinate the movement of your arms with the feet. Improved stability and a good connection with the ground occur as a byproduct of your relaxation and more upright posture – this is called developing a root.

The body can go through some quite dramatic changes after two or three months' practice, as the joints begin to open and articulate more freely. You may notice that the hips become more flexible, and the shoulder joints loosen, and this in turn can help the circulation.

It is quite likely that your coordination will be noticeably improved after the first two months or so of practising the t'ai chi form. Progress will be clearly recognized if you also practise some aspect of partner practice.

The sensation of *chi* may or may not be clear after one year of practice. Much depends upon the individual and the skill of the teacher to lead the student into the correct states of mind, as well as making the other influential factors clear and helping the student to put them into practice. The energy of *chi* is stimulated as you practise, even if you cannot actually feel the movement of the *chi* itself. You should find that within the first month of practice the amount of energy available to you during the day has improved as a result of your practice of the t'ai chi form.

You can expect your general feeling of well-being to be improved, even after the first class. Whether you are able to build upon this, or sustain the effects for longer periods, depends upon the amount of practice you do in your own time.

The first levels of t'ai chi chuan
An account of each of the different levels makes them appear as a series of linear steps, progressing from one to the next, but in reality they may overlap, and you will find that more advanced features of practice do manifest themselves occasionally during the earlier stages.

The first level of t'ai chi has already been mentioned; it is the habit most people have, when they begin a t'ai chi class, of opposing force with force. If you wish to avoid resisting your partner's energy you will have to learn to use the techniques of t'ai chi with a partner in a completely relaxed way, applying the four types of contact – touch, sticking, joining and following – together with some understanding of neutralizing energy and yielding. (Neutralizing energy is used with other techniques to turn the oncoming force of an adversary.) All of these techniques constitute the second level, called correct technique, and it is at this level that clear teaching is important. You will need to practise for some time to achieve competence at this level before your t'ai chi can progress to the next level, *jin* level. A good student can expect to have learnt the correct techniques within the first two years or so, but will need to practise for a further two years before the *jin* level begins to manifest itself.

Jin level is a general category, and includes the development of a number of different features of practice.

It corresponds to the development of *jin* for issuing energy with pushes, and with other similar techniques, and for responding to a partner's attack during neutralizing and yielding. The use of *jin* is so effective in its martial application that you are unlikely to be encouraged to develop its use with the conventional idea of striking with fist, elbow or foot. It is safer and easier to practise the methods of pushing and up-rooting (when the root of a person is severed and the push lifts him or her vertically upwards). It is whilst practising at this level that a student will learn to yield, in such a way that it is no longer possible to disturb his or her balance with any kind of push and the aggressor will lose his balance when he finds no resistance to the attack. All of these methods use *chi*, while making use of correct techniques. Some commentators refer to the *jin* level as the development of internal strength, but this term does not embrace the whole meaning.

These aspects of technique are fascinating, especially to those of us in the west who are not familiar with the workings of *chi*, but you do need to be patient, and wary of trying to develop advanced techniques before you have mastered the basics. Any attempt to miss out a stage of development will lead to the use of force to obtain results, and this defeats the purpose of studying t'ai chi.

HIGHER STATES OF T'AI CHI

The next level is called *chi* level. Now the t'ai chi expert has gained control of the *chi* to such an extent that he or she is able to project the energy outside the body, and so use the *chi* as an important component in pushing a partner. Whilst it is possible to cultivate the *chi* to be able to perform modest feats of this kind, it is rare in modern times for anyone to attain full mastery of this level. Traditionally the peak of achievement is demonstrated by the ability to draw a candle flame towards the hand from a distance of a few feet, and then to push it away and finally extinguish the flame completely. If you see a successful demonstration of the candle test then you can be sure that you have found a teacher with a good understanding of *chi* and the ability to use that knowledge. It is wise to remain sceptical if you see any other type of demonstration unless it also exhibits the use of *chi* upon an inanimate object.

Discussions about *chi* are full of controversy, and there is much debate as to the truth of some of the stories. This is particularly relevant at present, since, although t'ai chi has become more popular, there are few masters alive of a sufficiently high level to be able to demonstrate the power of *chi*. The stories, however, are plentiful.

The story of Chen Hsiu Feng

When Yang Lu-Shann became sick and died, his two sons, Yang Chen-Huo and Yang Ban-Huo, expected to become the head disciples. But Chen Hsiu Feng said that because the two sons had not practised when their father had been alive they did not deserve to take up the position, and that he, Chen Hsiu Feng, claimed the title as his own. The two sons went away in anger and began to study their father's notes and practise strenuously. Eventually, after three years, they felt ready to challenge Chen Hsiu Feng and so went to visit him.

When the brothers announced their claim Chen Hsiu Feng laughed because he had tricked them into practising, and had no intention of holding on to his position. He stretched out his hand and lifted a large armchair nearby using only the sticking energy of his palm, and put it down in front of Yang Chen-Huo and Yang Ban-Huo. The two brothers were shocked at this demonstration of *chi* as would we be.

It is difficult to believe stories like this when there are no individuals at this level of accomplishment living today. But we should be careful that our healthy scepticism does not close our minds to our own potential and limit our capabilities.

Mind, spirit and the natural way

The next levels after the *chi* level are mind, spirit, and natural way. Mind level is characterized by a very highly developed quality of sensitivity and lightness. Any response to a partner's attack is without any concern for *chi*, or *jin*, or any of the techniques belonging to the previous levels. The master responds with a thought and it is the same as if there were also the thought to act. Spirit indicates a type of awareness beyond ordinary consciousness – it has been described as being similar to the energy of decision – and natural way is a completely instinctive mastery of all the previous levels.

Human, earth and heaven stages

Cheng Man-Ching has used a different system for differentiating the levels of achievement. He has described the heaven, earth and human levels at which each have three degrees.

The human level relaxes the ligaments and tendons throughout the whole body in three stages, beginning from the shoulder to the wrist, then from the hip to the heel, and finally from the sacrum to the top of the head.

The earth level describes three stages of cultivation of *chi*. First, sinking the *chi* to the *tan tien*, then leading the *chi* into the arms and the legs and lastly moving the *chi* through the sacrum to the top of the head.

The highest level, called heaven, defines various degrees of sensitivity. The first degree is described as listening to, or feeling strength – to be able to use *jin* after you have detected and joined with your partner's *chi*. The second degree is called comprehension of *jin*, which refers to the subtle level of sensitivity achieved when a master is able to detect the very first manifestations of movement in an attacker's energy, before any physical movement occurs. The master is then able to coordinate the response perfectly. The final degree of achievement is called the omnipotent level, which corresponds to the level of spirit in the previous system. The t'ai chi definition of spirit is difficult to translate because it relates to a refined, or purified, form of *chi* which can be compared to mental energy or some type of power without any physical attributes. Spirit is expressed in the eyes; wherever the eyes concentrate, the spirit is able to reach and the *chi* follows. This level allows the master to move with lightning speed.

The five levels of the Wu style

The stages of development in the Wu style are clearly related to aspects of the t'ai chi syllabus as well as mapping out the internal changes. It takes about 10 years to progress through the various levels to the final stage of practice.

The first stage is called the mechanical level, when a student learns the correct way to stand in each posture of the form until precision is achieved. The next level, called unison of movement, is concerned with the roundness and smoothness of the movement itself; during this stage the applications are taught, together with an introduction to pushing hands. A student will also begin to practise specialized exercises, called *chi kung*, to develop the *chi*. Following on from this, at the level of mind control, the methods for leading the body with the mind are explained. The spear, broadsword and double-edged sword are started at this stage. At the fourth stage the emphasis is upon the cultivation of *chi*, and there are 24 *chi kung* forms which are special to the Wu style. The final level is called spirit, in which previous levels are integrated, improved and refined during practice.

SELF-DEFENCE ASPECTS OF T'AI CHI

If you are primarily interested in the self-defence aspect of t'ai chi, your patience is required. You will need to build up a strong connection with *chi*, together with an understanding of the principles of application and the necessary sensitivity and relaxation to be able to apply your understanding at speed. Your t'ai chi must become natural and instinctive. It makes sense to have an interest in the self-defence meaning of t'ai chi, but without too much desire to defeat anyone or deal with a real attack. In time you will be able to use t'ai chi principles to meet the effort of a partner to push you over.

Do not worry whether you are strong or weak, tall or short, as the principles for self-defence remain the same for everyone. You must learn to follow the intentions of your partner, and give up your own strength to feel clearly the force of your partner's attack. In t'ai chi you do not oppose a person's intentions but go with the force, and then take advantage of it when most of the power has been used up. When you first try to use these principles you will realize that it is not easy to avoid using force when you experience your partner pushing towards you. Success in t'ai chi depends upon your willingness to give up your fear of being pushed over, and learn to let go and relax. T'ai chi will engage your mind as well as help you learn to control your body.

There should be no strength in the hands. Some masters say that when pushing hands with a partner you should behave as if there is no one there in front of you; when you practise the solo form you should act as if there really is someone there. If you relax completely and your posture is correct, you will notice that the legs and the feet will feel relatively heavy compared with the arms and the upper body. You should avoid any grasping with the hands since this will deaden the lively quality of the upper body. The whole body should feel light, sensitive, and open.

When the time comes to return the attack, the energy is encouraged to flow from your feet through your body and into the hands. To be able to function in this way you will need to be rooted in the feet. Avoid using your shoulder strength to push your partner; feel instead that the push comes from the feet.

First you should learn the techniques for turning your partner's energy, and then, keeping your attention on the sensations of your partner's touch, develop an automatic application of the techniques. If you practise in this way you will be able to concentrate completely on your partner's energy and in the process forget yourself.

6
ADVICE FOR EFFECTIVE LEARNING

In the *Tao Te Ching*, Lao Tzu writes that, when a person pursues knowledge, and seeks to learn something, there is an accumulation of facts and knowledge; but when one practises the Tao, gradually there is a process of cutting away and a simplifying of life. The Taoist way of seeing the world becomes more rooted in the present. With a fresh vision, things are recognized as they are in the moment. The world appears as unified, harmonious and a totality, and the relative way of comparing the differences between separate aspects of the world is reduced day by day. Lao Tzu goes on to say that to attain the world one must remain free of desire and busy-ness, give up meddling and act in accord with the way of things.

When you go to your first t'ai chi class you are bound to have many expectations and preconceptions. These thoughts will only get in the way of actually meeting the experience with a completely open and present state of mind. Inevitably our minds colour the way we experience life, and distort any impressions we pick up of what is actually in front of us. The t'ai chi approach is a way of seeing what is there and using techniques to integrate the separate bits of ourselves into a more total way of being. In this way it is like meditation, but t'ai chi is active meditation and the principles are such that it is possible to apply them in everyday life. For example, if you are in a busy situation and everyone is rushing around, remember to centre yourself and relax; then you will be able to go with the flow of events without getting caught up in the anxiety of rushing, and yet still be able to act quickly and efficiently when the need arises.

THINKING AND FEELING

At the beginning the teacher will talk at length to explain the ideas surrounding t'ai chi, and lead you into your first t'ai chi movements; you will hear the advice, then will need to reflect upon the words and put them into practice. You will be thinking about what has been said, and thoughts will fill your head. But it is important to realize that t'ai chi relates very much to the feeling body – the world of feeling sensation – and the two activities of thinking and feeling cannot easily be experienced simultaneously. The principles and techniques of t'ai chi help you become much more involved with a feeling connection with yourself, but before you can reduce the amount of thinking you engage in you will need to be clear about how you are using your body in t'ai chi practice. So, as you learn the movements, the emphasis is on thinking and getting the actions correct; then, following on from this stage, use those techniques of movement to connect with the experience and feel what you are doing.

GETTING IT RIGHT, GETTING IT WRONG

You probably don't remember learning to walk and the way you went about achieving this basic skill. Children usually learn around the age of one; at this time language skills are limited and the whole idea of success and failure is undeveloped. A child will learn through trial and error, building upon successive experiences, from the struggle to stand upright and then beginning to take the first steps. There will be many times when the child falls down, but luckily it is unheard of for a child to give up trying. The so-called failures are really part of the process, and should be recognized as a valuable part of learning. When we mature as adults, very often there is a fear of failure and the mistakes we make when learning to do something are rarely valued; instead they are thought of as something to be eliminated. This attitude is inhibiting and blocks our readiness to be experimental and try different ways of doing things. The fear of making mistakes makes us tense. To relax in the t'ai chi class and during your own practice, you should be conscious that you are learning from your experience – and that includes the so-called mistakes.

If you are able to remember the postures easily and begin to feel confident that you are doing your t'ai chi well, then you will need to be careful that you do not become proud, since this can make it difficult to learn anything new. There is a balanced state of mind between feeling defeated by the mistakes you make and being inflated by your successes, and if you steer your mind towards this middle way then you will gradually calm the mind and deepen your relaxation on to a mental level.

THE INNER VOICE

You will find that t'ai chi can calm your mind very effectively as you practise the form slowly. When anyone begins to slow down the general busy-ness and activity of their daily life, a new inner world is revealed. At first the mental chatter of the thoughts seem to be unusually loud; a commentary on events, reactions to other people, thoughts about one's self, all seem to follow on in a stream of disjointed thoughts. Perhaps anxieties begin to enter your thoughts, ranging from emotional worries to more trivial concerns such as an overdue library book, or you begin to wonder if you turned the cooker off, and so on.

To begin to control this chatter and ease the tension of the mind, you will need to use a certain amount of skilful method. If you reject your thoughts, or try to push them away, you will only agitate the mind more than ever. If you are genuinely anxious about a particular topic, set aside some time to think about it or make a note of it and resolve to act on it later, then return to your practice. If the thoughts are more random, recognize and acknowledge them with an attitude of acceptance, and then return your attention to the movement. Acceptance is the attitude which will influence your mind positively and slowly bring you to calm states.

Sometimes there is a critical voice which feeds our negative thoughts about ourselves – 'I can't do this', 'I will never learn to relax', 'My t'ai chi is not very good'. We rarely stop for long enough to hear this voice and recognize what we are doing to ourselves. When the words are heard they are neutral – just sounds. It is the emotional content of the ideas behind the words which we respond to and begin to build up into a mood or state of mind. We talk ourselves into feeling a particular way. These negative thoughts are destructive and very restricting; they build up a poor image of ourselves which is very limiting. If you do catch yourself in a negative state, notice what is happening and decide not to get caught up in the mood; just listen to the words and then let go of the ideas behind the words. Words and thoughts are powerful, especially if you can generate the feeling and attitudes which go with them, and so it is a very good idea to take control and choose to listen to a positive mind.

CHANGING HABITS

Perhaps after you have learnt some postures in a class you will return home to find you can't be sure that you have remembered everything correctly. Should you practise when you may be forming a habit of moving in the wrong way?

The whole process of learning t'ai chi can be seen as one of learning to change habits, and so you need not feel that forming a wrong habit is something to be avoided. If you do practise a posture, but are uncertain whether it is performed in the correct way, even if it is incorrect it will still form the basis of learning it correctly in your next class.

If you are revising a posture you have just learnt in a class and you notice that there is something about the way you are doing it which needs some adjustment, do not stop in the middle of the movement; complete the posture and be aware of the way you are putting the actions together. Then perform the complete posture again without stopping, making the necessary changes. This way you will be practising to keep the continuity of the movement and looking at the whole, rather than breaking the posture down into component parts.

Habits form very quickly and require little effort in their formation. But to change a habit necessitates much more self awareness and discipline, to be in the moment and to feel free to choose to do things differently. Your presence of mind and awareness will be strengthened by your efforts to overcome any mistakes which have crept into your practice of the form.

T'ai chi is simple and easy to learn but the force of old habits make it seem difficult. If you can let go of your usual ways of being and use t'ai chi principles, then the feeling of struggle will gradually decrease and an assured feeling of relaxation will become the core of your practice.

DOING T'AI CHI CHUAN

When anyone begins to practise t'ai chi there is a feeling of doing the postures and making them happen. This is an attitude which we all adopt unconsciously when we are involved in directing things and trying to exert control over the outcome of events. The picture is one of struggle, with the emphasis on trying.

From a t'ai chi point of view this approach is unbalanced, and should be complemented with an attitude of acceptance, allowing the movements and experiences of t'ai chi to happen. Let your movement be influenced by the natural swing of free motion; allow the arms to hang from the shoulder joints; wait until the body is completely balanced before moving. These are examples of how you can cooperate with the natural ways of movement and begin to feel that t'ai chi itself makes the movements happen as much as you do. This can create a feeling of relief and put an end to the feeling of striving and trying too hard.

BEING PART OF A CLASS

There are ways to make the most of being in a class, which you might like to keep in mind. First, you should feel free to move around within the room, to find a good vantage point from which to see the teacher and any demonstration he or she may give. Feel free to ask the teacher to repeat any demonstration, or ask questions whenever they occur to you. A good teacher will be very appreciative of questions because they often have more significance than the student realized and can help to bring out new points of interest. If you feel a little inhibited in groups, then there is no need to pressurize yourself and ask questions before you are ready.

Being in the group is part of your t'ai chi, so remember to relax about the way you experience the class. Be aware that you don't always gravitate towards the same spot in the room – move around, sometimes stand near the front of the class, even if this makes you slightly uncomfortable, or be prepared to move to the back. If your class includes some partner practice, choose a different partner when you have the option so that you can have some variety.

It can be very useful to make notes during the class, or shortly afterwards, but this does not suit everyone.

If you feel tired physically, or you notice that your mind is becoming a little tight because of too much mental effort, then take a short rest – sit down if necessary. You will find that being more conscious of what you need at any particular time, and acting on it, will help you feel more centred and in touch with yourself.

Remember the class is specifically organized for you to learn t'ai chi. You need to find out how you, as an individual, can make the best use of it.

7
CHI AND T'AI CHI CHUAN

HOW IS *CHI* USED IN T'AI CHI?

It is a feature of t'ai chi that a student learns to develop
the imagination and strengthen the will, and with these
skills it is possible to develop a deeper level of relaxation
and gain some control of the mind. Just as a child will use
the imagination to create a world of play, the t'ai chi
player is able to create a positive state of mind and
influence the *chi*.

Normally it is not possible to feel *chi*. This is because
the *chi* is scattered throughout the body, and is unable to
flow freely when the joints and sinews are restricted. After
beginning t'ai chi the joints slowly open and the muscles
relax. A student learns to move in such a way that all the
joints remain open, and gradually, as the body becomes
coordinated and the mind develops some concentration,
the energy follows the idea of the action associated with
the application of the posture; the *chi* first collects and
then flows in response to the idea. The energy can then be
led to different parts of the body. The Chinese concept of
the mind includes the 'heart'. If a student is not sincere,
with a 'single heart', undistracted by other ideas, the *chi*
will not follow. To learn to move the *chi* during practice of
the form, a student learns to be present with what is
happening and yet at the same time to imagine the
meaning of the posture. For this to be most effective you
should believe as much as possible that the application is
actually being applied even though there is no adversary.
It is easy to see how t'ai chi became known as shadow
boxing.

THE BENEFITS OF CHI CULTIVATION

Any imbalance in the *chi* circulation is improved with practice of t'ai chi. For example, if the body is injured, this can cause an accumulation of *chi* in that particular part of the body, so causing an imbalance in the energy flow. Practising t'ai chi will encourage the normal distribution of energy, and the body will restore itself to a balanced state. T'ai chi provides gentle assistance to the *chi*, which always seeks to find a balance, even if it is not stimulated.

As the body begins to show signs of aging, hardness and stiffness increase, while softness and flexibility decrease. The deliberate use of t'ai chi to increase the amount of *chi* flowing freely in the body begins to revitalize the skin, helps to lubricate and open the joints and restore flexibility. The body will gain in strength as the *chi* accumulates and you begin to learn to control its use. With exercises in other sports and their associated use of strength, you will find that the power available to an individual begins to decline from 35 years onwards. In contrast, with t'ai chi and other systems of *chi* cultivation, the body may still be able to exert considerable strength in the 60s and 70s. For a younger person there is also a corresponding increase in vitality and strength.

The gentle movements of the forms stretch the body, releasing tension very effectively so that the whole body experiences a free flow of energy. The circulation of blood is also related to the flow of the *chi*, so problems of poor circulation can improve quite quickly with regular practice.

When the *chi* has been moving throughout the body there is often a strong sense of well-being, and the mind is more able to relax. The benefits which come from paying attention to the *chi* and moving it around the body are accumulative. Initially the feeling of *chi* is slight, but it increases when you become aware of its presence, as if it grows in response to being noticed.

HOW DO I LEARN TO FEEL *CHI*?

The benefits you will experience from your practice will increase quite dramatically once you have connected clearly with the feeling of *chi,* and so you should learn which t'ai chi techniques are important for *chi* cultivation. There are four main areas to consider – the mental attitude, sensitivity, breathing and the physical attitude.

The mental attitude

Some people are sceptical about the existence of *chi* and discount the possibility of feeling such a thing. By closing their minds to something which cannot be explained rationally they are also shutting themselves off from the benefits of such an experience. Many people analyse their experience so much that their thoughts prevent them from staying with the experience itself, and they become stuck with their thoughts. The thoughts have taken them away from the feeling. You should aim for a good connection with yourself on a feeling level, with an awareness of what is going on at the same time, but without that awareness getting in the way.

You will need to quieten your mind and learn to concentrate, in order to give yourself the right amount of mental focus, and then allow yourself to become sensitive to the more subtle sensations in the body.

Sensitivity

T'ai chi has been described as being like 'swimming in air'. For most of the time we move about freely, without taking too much notice of the air around us. Our movement is not restricted by open space and our eyes cannot see the air, even though it completely surrounds us. As a consequence of this, we ignore its subtle presence as we continue with our lives. However, when you begin your t'ai chi practice you will gradually become sensitive to the air in which we are immersed.

Bring your presence of mind to the hands, and try to feel the air as it passes over the skin when you move. Feel the more subtle touch of the air as it moves around the face. If you start to sensitize yourself in this way you will be able to feel the air quite easily, and it will begin to seem more dense. The air will start to feel more like water. At this stage your sensitivity has developed to the point where you will be able to feel *chi*, and it is a simple matter of remembering to continue your practice of the physical principles.

Learn to treat the air in a special way – this is called making use of the seemingly insubstantial. There is energy in the air, and if you become more familiar and aware in this way, you will be able to gather the energy as you practise.

Breathing
The breath is coordinated with the movement and the meaning of the posture. However, when you consider the order of what to practise first, you are well advised to leave the coordination of the breath until you have become familiar with the postures and their self-defence applications, although it can be good preparation to have the principles of breathing in the back of your mind so that when your teacher thinks the time is right you already know the method.

During the sinking yielding parts of the postures you should breathe in through the nose, and towards the end of your attacking movement you should breathe out, also through the nose. It is important not to empty completely at the end of exhaling because this will lose *chi*. At the end of the posture the *chi* is still maintained in the *tan tien*. The idea of *chi* is in the mind all the time and is gradually coordinated with the movement. The breath becomes finer, thinner, slower, longer and silent. The emphasis should be on the gradual and continuous nature of the practice. The breathing will become centred in the belly as you learn to relax and sink the *chi*.

The physical attitude
The body should be light and sensitive in all your t'ai chi practice. The spine will need to be held in a particular

position so that there are no restrictions to the flow of energy moving from the base of the spine up to the top of the head. The lower part of the spine is tucked under, and the head is held forward so that the chin is tucked in and the back of the neck is straightened. This is done in a very gentle way, otherwise it will restrict the flow. You should imagine that the whole body is suspended by a thread pulling up from the crown of the head. If you persevere with this technique not only will the spine be held open but, in time, any curvature of the spine will be lessened.

When practising t'ai chi there are times when the momentum of the movement, which begins at the feet, carries through into the upper body and causes it to twist slightly. This twist is natural but should not be permitted to turn the spine so far that there is an excessive distortion in the alignment of the spine. Think of a drinking straw – once it is twisted it becomes useless.

The front of the chest should feel loose or softened and the whole of the stomach area should feel soft and relaxed. This is achieved more easily if you avoid leaning backwards, which tightens the muscles down the front of the body. The strength of the body is located in the mid-back area before it is transmitted into the hands. The leverage from the ground which connects the whole-body energy to the hands is dependent upon the relationship between the feet and the position of the sacrum (the tailbone of the spine). You will need the guidance of your teacher to give you a practical demonstration of this point.

EXERCISES TO DEVELOP *CHI*

There are many exercises which are especially designed to stimulate and then move the internal energy of *chi* around the body. These exercises are called *chi kung* forms and they are each intended for a specific purpose, such as the improvement of health or the development of strength for martial art applications. Some *chi kung* exercises focus on one area of the body and others are more general in their effect.

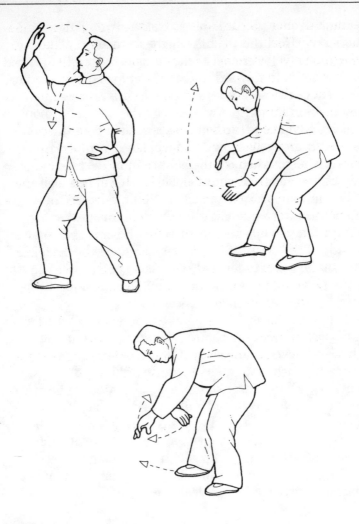

Movements from the flying crane *chi kung* exercise

Although many t'ai chi masters teach these methods for *chi* development, they are not strictly necessary if you practise the t'ai chi form correctly and carefully coordinate with the *chi*.

MORE ADVANCED STAGES

You will find that every principle of t'ai chi will be

meaningful once you are able to feel the body move as one unit and can feel the *chi* following your thought. The adjustments your teacher makes to your form will assist the flow of *chi* throughout the body, and when you can feel the effect of any corrections it will be easier for you to keep them in mind.

In the advanced stages of practice, t'ai chi becomes more of an internal art and you will learn as much from your own observations of the behaviour of *chi* inside the body as you will from your teacher's advice. It is as if the *chi* becomes an assistant teacher. You will be free to control the internal qualities of the body by moving the *chi*. At first, you will be able to empty the strength from one side of the body and make the other side of the body more substantial. Later your relaxation will enable the *chi* to sink down into the feet and you will begin to gain control of the *chi* throughout the length of the body, from the feet to the hands. This type of practice causes the concentration to improve and relaxation to deepen.

In the more advanced stages of practice it is important to keep the idea of *chi* in mind all the time.

8
THE T'AI CHI CHUAN CLASSICS

Past masters of t'ai chi have preserved their knowledge and experience in short cryptic writings, which are easy to memorize, and yet manage to encapsulate many of the essential principles. These classics have been handed down from master to student over many generations, even though the identity of some of the authors may have been lost. The meaning is often open to argument and interpretation; the Chinese language has a very different grammatical structure from English and there can be no direct translation, since each phrase in Chinese can be translated in several different ways. The translator must also have a similar experience to the original author in order to give an adequate commentary.

There follows a selection of some of the t'ai chi classics which will be useful, particularly at the beginning of your t'ai chi studies.

CHANG SAN-FENG'S ADVICE

Chang practised t'ai chi during the 14th century and he wrote that:

- In every movement the entire body should be light and agile, and all of its parts connected like a string of pearls.

The whole body should be moved without any restriction to the internal energy and without any unnecessary tension. It will then be possible to unify the movements, using the energy of *chi* to connect the separate parts of the

body – like a thread which links separate pearls. The
lightness comes from being responsive, alert and sensitive
to the most delicate touch; if someone were to press any
part of the body they would find no resistance. With this
kind of lightness comes agility.

- The postures should be without faults, without
  deficiency or excess, and without any discontinuities.

The shapes of the postures should be complete when
considered as a whole. The roundness expressed in the
body should not be restricted or cramped so that there is a
'deficiency', or, to consider the other extreme, there
should be no over-extension or 'excess' in any direction.

The movement during your practice should be
expressed by the whole body and should be continuous.
For example, when pushing, the various elements of the
body are coordinated with the movement. The shift of
weight, turn of the hips and movement of the arms all
occur at the same time. When any one of these elements
stops moving, then the whole body should stop or,
conversely, when any one element is in motion then the
whole body should be in motion – the movement is
'without discontinuities'.

Another classic by Wang Tsung-Yueh explains that the
energy of t'ai chi should be expressed like drawing silk
from a cocoon. This image refers to the nature of silk when
it is pulled. If the silk is pulled too suddenly it will snap; if
there is hesitation or the action is uneven the silk will
snag. When pulling silk the speed must be even and
continuous.

- The energy (*jin*) is rooted in the feet, develops in the
  legs, is directed by the waist, and expressed by the
  fingers. The connection from the feet, through the legs
  to the waist, must act as one unit so that when
  advancing and retreating you obtain a good
  opportunity and a superior position.

The root is more than just a simple physical connection with the ground, and it comes into being when there is a feeling of relaxing through the feet – literally into the ground.

This feature of t'ai chi needs more detailed explanation and some exploration on your part to grasp the full meaning. If you look at your hand you can see the shape clearly delineated; the outline is distinct and there is no doubt where the hand finishes and the air begins. Now, close your eyes and feel the hand and try to get some clear idea of the shape. The boundary between where the hand finishes and the air begins is by no means clear. The sensation of the hand has a completely different shape from the one we so clearly see with our eyes. It is as if the feeling body is a different body from the one we see, and that the shape of the feeling body is much less bounded by edges – it is possible to feel beyond the boundaries of the skin.

When we explore the sensation of the feet in contact with the ground we can notice the same experience. The ground is clearly flat, yet the sensation of the foot in contact with the flatness of the ground does not feel like a clear boundary. There are areas where the foot feels as though it extends through into the ground, and places where the hardness of the ground is more apparent. The main point here is that the boundaries are not as clearcut as we may have assumed. The mind has a habit of not feeling what is actually happening, and holds on to the idea that the boundaries exist, even when, after closer examination, they cannot be found in experience.

If you relax all the bones and muscles in the feet and allow the sensation of the feet to settle through the ground, you will begin to find your connection with the ground has developed, making you feel much more stable and rooted. Cheng Man-Ching said that the feet should be as if they are glued to the ground. He used the image of a camel's foot settling into the desert sand, and said that when you practise you must get firm connections. The feet should feel heavy and the upper body feel light.

To make the energy of *jin* effective it must come from prolonged practice of the form, linking every movement from the feet. The energy is rooted in the feet, developed from the use of the legs, is then directed by the waist and is allowed to flow through the upper body and be expressed in the hands. From this explanation it is easy to see why there should not be any break in the continuity from the foot to the fingers. When the *jin* is activated in this way and the body acts as one unit, it is possible to be well coordinated with a partner's attack, either when retreating or moving forward, so that no opportunity will be lost.

Many of the same points are restated in this next classic, with a new emphasis.

- The substantial and insubstantial must be clearly distinguished. Every part of the body has both a substantial and insubstantial aspect at any particular time and the whole of the body has an insubstantial and a substantial aspect. All the joints of the body are to be threaded together without a single break.

What is the meaning of substantial and insubstantial? They are both commonly used words to describe internal qualities which you will begin to feel as you practise t'ai chi. If you are pushed on your right side and you respond sensitively so that you keep contact with your partner's hand, but at the same time offer no resistance, then you have made your right side change from substantial at the moment before you felt the push to insubstantial at the moment of moving sensitively to accommodate your partner's force. When the right side of the body changes in this way to become insubstantial, the left side of the body also changes and becomes substantial. This can be compared to going through some revolving doors; you push one side of the door and this begins to rotate, allowing you through the opening, but you must not hesitate in the middle because there is another revolving door following close behind. When a t'ai chi expert becomes insubstantial on one side, in order to yield to a partner's force, the other side becomes substantial and can deliver an attack, similar to the revolving door. This technique also functions with any attack on a part of the body. For example, if the elbow is attacked, this can be made insubstantial and the wrist and hand can then

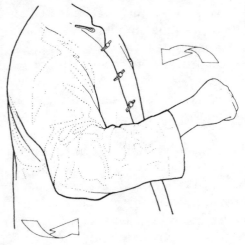

The elbow yields to the force of an attack

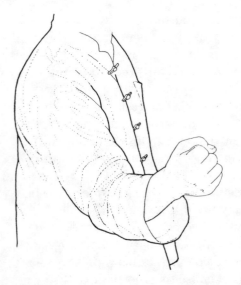

The fist returns the force of the original attack using a circular response

A folding technique

become substantial. This time a better analogy would be a child's seesaw – as the elbow gives way, the wrist comes forward, with a pivot point somewhere in between. The t'ai chi term for this technique is folding energy.

Another related idea is the transition from full to empty and empty to full. This can be demonstrated clearly when stepping. The weight should be clearly balanced in one foot before taking a step. The foot with the weight in it is called full and the other leg is empty. If you practise stepping only when the leg is completely empty you will be able to move in a very fluid way and without any loss of balance.

These changes from insubstantial to substantial, and so on, must be clearly defined and should not be muddled or incomplete. It is important to practise every shift of your weight without doubt, and to be sure that you are balanced in one foot before taking a step or lifting your foot to kick. Your understanding of the changes that occur in the body will develop with your experience of pushing hands and other partner exercises.

Some of these classics seem to relate exclusively to the martial art aspect of t'ai chi, with little relevance to other motives for practice. However, you should realize that t'ai chi is an internal practice and it is only through understanding the function of the techniques that you will be able to use them for more peaceful purposes. The self-defence application is the means and not the end.

- T'ai chi chu'an is also called long boxing because it is like a long river which rolls on ceaselessly. Ward off, roll back, press, push, pull, split, elbow stroke, and shoulder stroke are the eight trigrams.
- Step forward, step back, look left, look right, and central equilibrium are the five elements.
- Ward off, roll back, press, push, are Heaven, Earth, Water, and Fire and are the four cardinal directions. Pull, split, elbow, shoulder stroke are Wind, Thunder, Lake and Mountain and are the four diagonal directions.

- Step forward, step back, look left, look right, and central equilibrium are metal, wood, water, fire and earth.
- All together these make up the thirteen postures.

Why is t'ai chi called long boxing? Because the form is continuous from start to finish, without any break; it is like the unbroken line of a circle. There were originally 13 postures as described in this classic, but afterwards many teachers taught more and the long form of Yang Cheng-Fu's day contained many repeated sequences. However, if you can understand the form and function of the 13 postures you will discover that you understand the essence of all postures.

This classic explains the relationship between t'ai chi and the trigrams of the *I Ching* or *Book of Changes*. It names the individual postures and relates them to the eight directions. The eight postures are the eight basic self-defence applications, and their relationship to the directions can be explored when you practise the *da lu* exercise with a partner.

T'ai chi theory explains how the primal state of *wu chi* gives rise to t'ai chi, and how this then produces yin and yang – the two polar opposites – which interact to give the four phases and then the eight trigrams. These trigrams combine to form the 64 hexagrams described in the *I Ching*. The progressive divisions are made so that all the various possible states can be included in their subtle complexity within the theory, and yet all this complexity has its origin in the simple and basic relationship between yin and yang.

Extreme yang gives way, by a process of gradual change, to become extreme yin, but even at the most extreme state the yang will contain the seed of yin, and in the same way the final state of yin will have the seed of yang. These cyclical changes express the continuous processes of creation and destruction. The five different steps can be explained in terms of creation and destruction, using the symbolism of the Taoist elements.

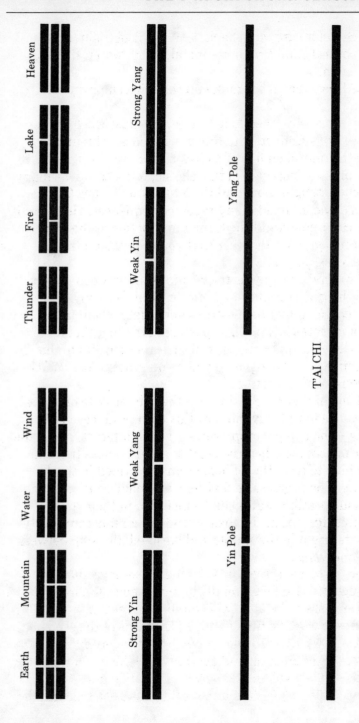

T'ai chi produces eight trigrams

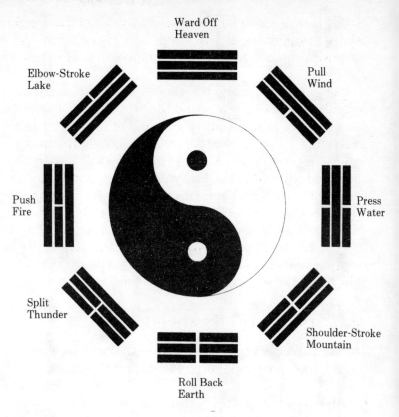

Chang San-Feng's arrangement of the eight basic postures

Step forward has a vigorous, fierce quality and so corresponds to fire. Central equilibrium has the nature of stability and corresponds to earth. If you step forward with stability, there is no doubt or uncertainty and it is easy to accomplish your goal. This is fire producing earth. Look left has the attribute of hardness and corresponds to metal. During a step to the left, at the same time you punch with the right fist, keeping your stability. This is earth producing metal. Step back uses the quality of softness, and corresponds to water. The hardness of look left gives support to the attribute of water. The softness of step back is not extreme since it contains the idea of moving back and so is connected with the idea of strength

– this is represented by water producing wood. Look right relates to strength and is represented by wood. Step forward with wood balancing it produces fire. The cycle is complete.

The symbolism which the Taoist's use to explain the balance of forces in nature and the processes of change are not necessary to the study of t'ai chi, but they do give an interesting flavour to the search for ways to harmonize with conflicting forces. Much of this knowledge is already contained within t'ai chi, and you will find that as you practise the form and build up your experience of partner techniques, your reflection on the principles will bring its own insight into the processes of change. It is not helpful to study too much on a theoretical level before you have a store of experience, but to go back to the theory later will help you make sense of your experience.

WANG TSUNG-YUEH'S ADVICE

The classics of Wang chosen for this section offer advice about how to adopt the correct posture for t'ai chi.

• An insubstantial energy draws the head upward. The *chi* is sunk to the *tan tien.*

When you begin t'ai chi there is a great deal of emphasis on relaxation and sinking, with careful attention given to the way you take steps and keep your balance. This can begin to make the body feel heavy, especially if the head is allowed to slump forward and the chest becomes constricted. Although the primary feeling is one of sinking and the downward flow of energy is important, in this classic we are advised at the same time to feel a light and active energy at the top of the head. It is as if the crown of the head is very gently suspended by a thread, drawing the head into an upright position with the chin tucked in slightly. The back of the neck becomes straightened, allowing the circulation to the head to improve which, together with a sense of awareness at the top of the head, will draw the 'spirit of vitality' to the top of the head and increase alertness.

The *chi* is sunk down to the *tan tien* (the energy centre below the navel) and then to the feet. The alignment of the body is experienced both as an upward flow of energy from the feet going through the tailbone up to the head, and as a downward flow through the front of the body to the *tan tien* and into the feet.

You will be able to lead the *chi* down to the *tan tien* after your contact with energy has become familiar and you are able to relax.

- There should be no tilting or leaning in any direction. Suddenly disappear, suddenly appear.

This classic offers uncompromising advice; there should be no leaning in any direction. For the body to be balanced it must be aligned completely upright, so that the forces of gravity move through the upper body and are then transmitted through the legs down into the feet. You should pay special attention to the relationship between the sacrum, or tailbone, and the ground – the sacrum is maintained in a vertically upright position. Every part of the posture should be level and straight, and you should think of vertical and horizontal planes to help simplify the idea. This helps the body weight to pass through the centre of the feet, rather than being pushed to the edges, causing the feet to roll and lose their stability. When the body is upright the muscles in the back are not used to prevent the body from slumping forward; the front of the body is also able to remain relaxed if there is no tendency to lean backwards. The perfectly balanced body is able to be very sensitive in its responses to a partner's attack, and it is in this way that we are able to 'suddenly disappear, suddenly appear'.

- The fundamental point is to forget oneself and to follow others. Many misunderstand this point and give up the near for the far. This means that a slight error

can cause a thousand-mile deviation from the path.
The student should be careful to discriminate the
correct way.

This principle touches on the most profound teaching of
t'ai chi. The meaning is most clearly understood when
considered during your practice of t'ai chi with a partner.
When you make contact with your partner's touch, you
decide that you will allow your partner to move first and
then follow your partner's intention. For example, if your
partner moves towards you with a push, you feel the
weight and the direction of the force and then begin to
move at the same time, following the direction of your
partner's push without resisting or breaking contact. At
the same time as making this response, you introduce a
turning circle and gently lead your partner's energy away
from your body. During the use of this technique you
must give up your own strength and concentrate fully on
the actions of the adversary. This means that you forget
your usual sense of self, and your movement will be well
coordinated and agile.

If you try to take the initiative at the outset in order to
determine the outcome of an event, you have given up
being in the present moment and your mind will be
reaching into the future to the idea of how you want things
to be. This causes you to ignore the actions of your
partner, and your movements become clumsy and badly
timed – inevitably you end up using force.

Wang then gives a warning reminder that, if you set off
in the wrong direction by even the slightest amount, you
will miss your chosen destination by a huge margin. So
Wang stresses the importance of being wary at the
beginning to ensure that your understanding will lead to
further insights.

• Step like a cat

When a cat is uncertain whether the ground is firm it
steps very lightly, placing the foot down without any shift

of balance. If the ground proves to be solid enough, the shift of weight then follows. A t'ai chi expert will place the foot before moving the centre of gravity, keeping the body perfectly balanced during the step. This is practised slowly and deliberately at the beginning, but it soon becomes a habit to be stable at all times, whether moving quickly or slowly. Most people walk with the weight falling forward on to the stepping leg, which lands with a thump, whereas the step of a cat is silent and full of poise.

9
THE ESSENTIAL PRINCIPLES FOR A BEGINNER

There can be many positive benefits from learning something about t'ai chi before finding a class, but you do need to remind yourself that at the beginning of your t'ai chi study the application of the theory should be kept to a minimum and the emphasis placed on your practice. It is when you have built up a store of practical knowledge that you will find it invaluable to reflect upon the classics and the theory of t'ai chi, to stimulate your imagination and inspire you to further effort.

Learning t'ai chi is a process of self-discovery and in a short time you will learn to connect internally with the sensations inside your body and experience simple acts like stepping in a much more conscious way. After you have learnt a posture and no longer have to think about it in order to practise your t'ai chi, you should focus your attention on the internal experience and learn to relax the body. First you must get the outside to look correct and then the inside will gradually begin to be more meaningful.

RELAX

Relaxation is central to t'ai chi. So much of our everyday life produces stress, and you will constantly need to remind yourself to relax. Learning to let go and relax is a creative process – the unconscious holding on prevents our habit from changing easily, and you will need to experiment with different images or ways in which you experience your body in order to free yourself from habit.

For example, to let the arms hang you must allow them to feel heavy, to swing freely and perhaps to bump gently against the body. At first the arms feel heavy as they relax, but the practice of t'ai chi opens the shoulder joints, and the *chi*, flowing into the arms, will make them feel light. Or, if you become aware that your shoulders are raised, simply remember to let them drop. During the day, every time you notice that your shoulders are raised, persist with your effort to relax them. At first you will forget for most of the time, and only occasionally remember to let them down, but things will gradually change until your shoulders will remain relaxed almost all the time and instead you will notice the few times in the day that they lift. This is a slow process, but the value of relaxation is so easily recognized that you should feel inspired to remember, whether you practise t'ai chi on a regular basis or not. Remembering to relax is not only physically beneficial but also increases mental awareness and presence of mind.

It is possible to relax in the wrong way if your mind is not alert. For example, be aware of the different possible ways that the hands can be relaxed, and this will give you an insight into how to adjust the whole body. If the hand is held with the fingers curling then this suggests that there is insufficient alertness; you should hold the finger joints open, but at the same time be careful not to make the hands too stiff.

CENTRAL EQUILIBRIUM AND THE *TAN TIEN*

Central equilibrium is the t'ai chi term given to the upright balanced posture which is an important feature of every t'ai chi position. This is one of the most important principles to attend to, especially at the beginning of your studies. When the body is erect the downward gravitational forces move easily through the body, and there is a sensation of sinking as the *chi* is encouraged to move down the front of the body to the *tan tien*. The *tan tien* is the body's centre of gravity, located in the abdomen, close to the navel. The relationship between the idea of central equilibrium and the *tan tien* is important. Some awareness remains in the *tan tien* at all times, whilst the waist acts as a pivot point for all the movements and directs the expression of the energy into the upper body and the hands. The ease with which this flow of energy can pass from the legs into the hands is also dependent upon the alignment of the spine.

When you first try to bring your feeling connection down to the *tan tien* you may find this difficult. You may find your sense of contact gets stuck in some other place and you cannot feel any real sensation at the point of the *tan tien*. If you practise the following simple exercise this should improve. Place the middle fingers of both hands over the *tan tien* (which is three finger-widths below the navel) and rest them gently but firmly in contact with your body. Close your eyes and then become aware of your breathing. On an inbreath take your thoughts down to the sensation of touch, where your fingers contact the *tan tien*. Keep your awareness of the feeling sensation down with your *tan tien* for about five minutes and then on an outbreath release your contact with the *tan tien* and open your eyes. With regular practice this will improve the ease with which you can connect with the lower part of the body.

COORDINATING THE WHOLE BODY

As you learn to relax and begin to be more aware of the legs and waist when you move, you will find that the upper body will tend to be more resistant to relaxation and continues to move independently because this habit is so strong. However, when you have learned the correct techniques, the whole body may be set in motion from the slightest pull on one hair of your head.

Before you reach this level you will need to be especially aware of the movements that begin with a sensation of pushing from the feet, which in turn affects the hips, which then transmit the energy into the arms and hands.

To help keep this in mind, remember that when one part of the body moves, the whole body moves. Although you will be encouraged by your teacher to practise the whole posture, including the arm movements, it is a good idea to spend some of your practice time paying special attention to the legs and the waist, without too much concern for what the arms are doing.

IN T'AI CHI THE ARMS DO NOT MOVE

Cheng Man-Ching tells a story about how one night he dreamed that he had broken his arms and was practising the form without being able to move them, except as part of his body movement. The next day in his partner-practice with his senior students his t'ai chi had improved so much that everyone was curious to discover his new secret. The dream had inspired him to relax his arms

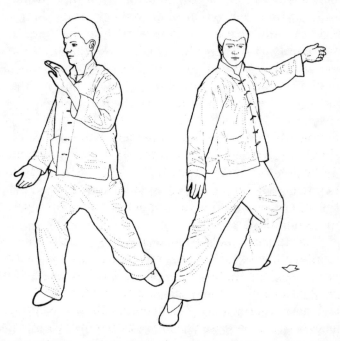

When pushing, the shift of weight from the back foot is coordinated with the pushing hand

completely and to use his body and waist to move them.

The arms and the body should move as one unit, but if you take this advice to an extreme you will be in danger of becoming too stiff; it is important to be careful that you allow some freedom in the shoulder-joints, so that the arms are loose as well as being well connected with the body. The hands and the feet do move, but the point here is that they do not move independently.

The hips are kept loose, in spite of the fact that you are directing your arm movements with the turns of the waist. There is a technique to keep in mind which will help you loosen the muscles around the hips and allow some freedom in the hip joint. When moving the weight from the back foot forward into the front foot, the moving force comes from a push from the back foot. For example, if you are standing with your left foot in front of the right, with your weight centred in the back foot, to begin the forward movement you will need to make the left hip feel very loose and relaxed so that when you begin to push from the right foot the weight moves forward with the hips straight. In a similar way, when the weight is moving from the front foot into the back foot, it is the front foot which pushes the body back. In every shift of weight in t'ai chi there is only one leg which provides the moving force. If there is strength in both legs at the same time, this is called being double weighted; this is a fundamental mistake and should be avoided right from the start. A common habit for beginners when shifting the weight is to push from one foot to only a limited extent so that there is also a pull into the other foot, and it is this tendency which produces tension in the hips.

The stances should be long enough so that there is some mental effort to gather your momentum when you step, but not so long that there is any physical struggle. If you are comfortable with a short stance and then feel awkward when you lengthen your stride to the optimum length, this is because you are resisting the openness of the more open posture and this resistance produces tension. It is worth exploring this point, with your teacher's supervision, to get the right balance in your practice.

INVEST IN LOSS

If you are already quite strong when you begin t'ai chi it can become something of a handicap if you are unwilling to give up your ordinary strength in order to develop t'ai chi strength. This is the meaning of the advice to invest in loss. If you already consider yourself weak then you will find it easier to avoid using force, because you have less strength to relinquish.

Another meaning to the phrase is that you should not take shortcuts in order to satisfy your urge to make rapid progress. If you are greedy, nothing is thoroughly chewed. Concentrate your efforts on becoming soft and relaxed, and connect with the energy of *chi.*

WHY IS SOFTNESS IMPORTANT?

The use of softness in t'ai chi has a number of different explanations. The Taoists recognize that all things become stiff and hard with the onset of death, whereas all living things are soft and flexible. When you practise t'ai chi you are making the decision to vitalize your energy by being in harmony with the qualities of the *chi.* There is a return to the bodily attributes of an infant. The energy of *chi* is associated with softness, and so when you choose to become soft you are attuning your mind and body to connect with yourself on a more subtle level.

When an attacker comes towards you with hard physical force, your response should be to use an equal amount of softness so that you can act in a harmonious way and find the correct technique to balance your adversary's attack before making your own. The t'ai chi master is able to use internal strength to produce hardness at the appropriate moment, but for health it is not necessary to develop this technique.

SOME FINAL WORDS OF ADVICE

When you have found a suitable teacher and have joined a class, then you should make time in your daily routine to practise. It is not a good idea to practise for a long session on one day and then to neglect your practice the next day; try to find some continuity, even if this means you settle for a shorter period on a more regular basis. Cheng Man-Ching advised his students to look at the heavens moving very gradually. They do not decide to move a little more, nor do they jump. The movement of the stars and planets is regular and predictable.

Seek for an open mind so that you can appreciate your experiences. We are all too quick to limit ourselves; we should encourage each other to be more positive and explore our potential. Try to keep to the truth and practise sincerely with true feeling. T'ai chi chuan can reveal many things if we allow it to influence us and feel that it acts upon us rather than that we are the ones in control and 'doing' t'ai chi.

GLOSSARY

chi (or ***ch'i***) The vital energy of all living beings; breath or the energy of the breath. There are two types of *chi* – prenatal *chi* and postnatal *chi*. You are born with prenatal *chi* which comes from your parents. After birth this is gradually consumed, and you begin to replace it with postnatal *chi* developed from food or air.

chi kung A specialized exercise to increase the amount of *chi* circulating in the body and to cultivate specific effects such as improved health or strength for martial application.

conception vessel Also known by the Chinese name *jen mai*. It is one of the eight extra meridians, and runs from the perineum, upwards along the centre line of the front of the body, over the throat, to a point just below the lower lip.

da lu This means 'long rollback', and is the name given to an active exercise performed with a partner, emphasizing the postures which comprise the four corners and the four directions.

follow When your partner moves, you follow whilst keeping sticking contact. Each action which the adversary makes is mirrored with an appropriate response, without allowing any gap or separation of energy to open up.

force When trying to overcome resistance by using superior strength, it is called using force. When applying force the muscles bind together into a rigid structure, using one set of muscles pulling against another set. The Chinese call the ordinary use of muscular strength *li*. In t'ai chi chuan it is important to avoid using this type of strength and learn to develop *jin*.

four corners The name given to the four postures pull-down, split, elbow and shoulder-stroke.

four directions The name given to the four postures ward-off, roll-back, press and push.

governor vessel Also known by the Chinese name *du mei*; it is one of the eight extra meridians. It runs from the tailbone, up the spine, to the roof of the mouth.

I Ching The *Book of Change*. It is considered to be the oldest of the Chinese classics and is dated around fourth century BC. It explains the fundamental principles of change from a Taoist point of view.

internal strength The Chinese term for this is *jin*. It is one of the main objectives in the development of t'ai chi chuan. There are many different types of *jin*, some of which can be used sensitively for detecting a partner's strength and others for turning a partner's force or striking. It is said that *jin* is able to produce its power from the sinews rather than from the muscles.

jin (or ***chin***) The Chinese term for internal strength or intrinsic energy.

join When your partner pushes you or tries to make a sticking contact, you join by feeling their mind's intention, keeping contact yourself but presenting your partner from sticking to you.

meridian The pathway followed by the *chi* as it moves around the body.

spirit A level of awareness beyond mental consciousness.

sticking To stick is to keep continuous contact with a partner, maintained at a point of contact.

t'ai chi, wu chi *Wu chi* is the primordial state, before any beginning. When there is any movement away from this undifferentiated state, this is called *t'ai chi* and gives rise to the world of dual opposites of yin and yang. The practice of t'ai chi chuan is a way of finding harmony within the processes of change and learning to understand *t'ai chi.* (One must be careful not to get confused when reading or hearing the common shortening of t'ai chi chuan to t'ai chi – this is not the same as the philosophical idea.)

tan tien (lower)   A centre of energy located three finger-widths below the navel. During t'ai chi chuan the *chi* is allowed to sink to the *tan tien.*

Taoism   A philosophy and religion whose followers were united in their aim to seek a Tao or Way. The early Chinese character for Tao showed a head, together with the sign for going, but the meaning of Tao for the Taoists became charged with deep spiritual and philosophical meaning, almost impossible to translate. It became a symbol for the underlying order in nature.

yielding   This is a quality which was valued by the early Taoists. In the *Tao Te Ching*, written by Lao Tzu, he says that 'The highest good is like that of water. The goodness of water is that it benefits the thousand creatures, yet itself does not wrangle, but is content with the places that all other men disdain. It is this that makes water so near to the Tao.' Water is yielding because it always seeks the lower position, and becomes great as a result; like a great river or sea gains from the smaller streams by being lower so that the streams flow into them. The t'ai chi master takes the lower position when faced with force and adopts the soft yielding character of water.

yin and yang   The Chinese characters for yin and yang are connected with darkness and light. The image of yin is a shadow behind a hill or clouds, while the character for yang has slanting sun-rays or a person holding a symbol of Heaven. They represent the fundamental opposites of the female (yin) and the male (yang) characteristics.

REFERENCE SECTION

BIBLIOGRAPHY

T'ai chi books

Y.K. Chen, *Tai-Chi Ch'uan*, Newcastle Publishing, USA, 1979.

Cheng Man-Ching and Robert Smith, *T'ai Chi*, Charles Tuttle, USA, 1982.

Cheng Man-Ching, *Cheng Tzu's Thirteen Treatises on T'ai Chi Chuan* (trans. Benjamin Pang Lo), North Atlantic Books, USA, 1985.

Jou Tsung Hwa, *The Tao of T'ai-Chi Chuan*, Charles Tuttle, USA, 1980.

T.T. Liang, *T'ai Chi for Health and Self-Defense*, Vintage Books, New York, USA, 1977.

Douglas Wile (compiled and translated from Chinese), *T'ai Chi Touchstones: Yang Family Secret Transmissions*, Sweet Chi Press, USA, 1983.

Wu-style classics can be obtained from Gary Wragg (see teachers and organizations below).

T'ai chi philosophy

Thomas Cleary (trans.), *The Taoist I Ching*, Shambala, 1986.

Lao Tzu, *The Complete Works of Lao Tzu. Tao Teh Ching and Hua Hu Ching* (trans. and elucidation by Ni Hua-Ching), The Shrine of the Eternal Breath of Tao, USA, 1982.

Man-jan Cheng, *Lao Tzu: 'My words are very easy to understand.' Lectures on the Tao Teh Ching* (trans. Tam C. Gibbs), North Atlantic Books, USA, 1981.

Joseph Needham, *The Shorter Science and Civilisation in China: 1*, Cambridge University Press, 1980.

Richard Wilhelm (trans.), *The I Ching or Book of Changes*,
Routledge & Kegan Paul, London, 1969.

TEACHERS AND ORGANIZATIONS

The t'ai chi schools listed here have, as their main
instructor, either a recognized master of t'ai chi or an
instructor who has studied extensively with such a
master.

London
John Kells
British T'ai Chi Chuan Association
7 Upper Wimpole Street
London W1
01-935 8444.

Gary Wragg
Wu's T'ai Chi Chuan Academy
London Centre of Wu Style T'ai Chuan
PO Box 1724
London W9 1YQ

Chu King-Hung
The International T'ai Chi Chuan
People's Hall
No. 8 Oriental Arts Studio
91–7 Freston Road
London W11
01-229 2900

John Eastman
The Jun Chi T'ai Chi Chuan Association
55 Old Town
London SW4
01-727 4427

Adrian Murray
12 Wray Crescent
London N4 3LP
071-281 5535

Bristol
Alan Peck
Natural Way T'ai Chi School
22 Withleigh Road
Knowle
Bristol BS4 2LQ
0272 771733

Sheffield
David Barrow
Wu Style T'ai Chi
161 Long Lane
Sheffield S11 7TX

Wales
Richard Farmer
Rising Dragon T'ai Chi
5 St John Street
Penarth
Cardiff CF6 1DN
0222 707443

Barbara Richter
The Town Hall
Llanidloes
Powys

West of England
Angus Clark
Devon T'ai Chi
Mill Farm
East Week
South Zeal
EX20 2QB

USA

Benjamin P. Lo
Universal T'ai Chi Chuan Association
2901 Clement St
San Francisco
CA 94121

Steve Brit
Detroit
Michigan
Can be contacted through Wu Kwong Yu in Canada.

Jou Tsung Hwa
T'ai Chi Farm
PO Box 630
New Milford
NY 10959

T'ai Chi
Wayfarer Publications
PO Box 26156
Los Angeles
CA 90026
Catalogue of T'ai Chi books for sale included in each issue.

Canada

Wu Kwong Yu
140 D'Arcy St
Toronto
Canada M5T 1G6

INDEX

Alan Peck became interested in Chinese philosophy whilst studying art in London and Hull. He was a primary school teacher for 7 years before studying t'ai chi with John Kells, the first westerner to be recognized as a Master by the Chinese T'ai Chi Chuan Association.

In 1983, having been the top student at the British T'ai Chi School, Alan Peck moved to Bristol to establish the Natural Way T'ai Chi School, and received final instruction from Dr Chi Chiang-Tao.

Alan Peck also practises meditation, and is a trustee of the Lam Rim Bristol Trust, which has a centre for Mahayana Buddhism.

AN INTRODUCTION TO
<u>AIKIDO</u>
Jon Pearson

Aikido – the way of Harmony – is an ingenious and non-aggressive system of self-defence in which an unprovoked attack is neutralised by pinning or throwing techniques, causing the minimum of harm to the assailant.

Second Dan Jon Pearson provides a fresh insight into the essential principles of this graceful Japanese martial art. He explains the profound influence of the founder Morihei Ueshiba, how Aikido redefines power and force, and how the practical techniques are designed to promote harmony, spiritual fulfilment and the peaceful resolution of conflict.

An indispensable guide to all students, this book covers:
* History and philosophy
* Practical aspects of training
* Weapons practice
* Aikido organisations

All Optima books are available at your bookshop or newsagent, or can be ordered from the following address:
  Little, Brown and Company (UK) Limited,
  P.O. Box 11,
  Falmouth,
  Cornwall TR10 9EN.

Alternatively you may fax your order to the above address. Fax No. 0326 376423.

Payments can be made as follows: cheque, postal order (payable to Little, Brown and Company) or by credit cards, Visa/Access. Do not send cash or currency. UK customers and B.F.P.O. please allow £1.00 for postage and packing for the first book, plus 50p for the second book, plus 30p for each additional book up to a maximum charge of £3.00 (7 books plus).

Overseas customers including Ireland, please allow £2.00 for the first book plus £1.00 for the second book, plus 50p for each additional book.

NAME (Block Letters) ....

....

ADDRESS ....

....

....

☐ I enclose my remittance for _____

☐ I wish to pay by Access/Visa Card

Number ⬚⬚⬚⬚⬚⬚⬚⬚⬚⬚⬚⬚⬚⬚⬚⬚

Card Expiry Date ⬚⬚⬚⬚